I0113242

OVERLOOKED

OVERLOOKED

Counselor Insights for the Unspoken Issues in Black American Life

LaVerne Hanes Collins

ROWMAN & LITTLEFIELD
Lanham • Boulder • New York • London

Published by Rowman & Littlefield
An imprint of The Rowman & Littlefield Publishing Group, Inc.
4501 Forbes Boulevard, Suite 200, Lanham, Maryland 20706
www.rowman.com

86-90 Paul Street, London EC2A 4NE

Copyright © 2024 by LaVerne Hanes Collins

All rights reserved. No part of this book may be reproduced in any form or by any electronic or mechanical means, including information storage and retrieval systems, without written permission from the publisher, except by a reviewer who may quote passages in a review.

British Library Cataloguing in Publication Information Available

Library of Congress Cataloging-in-Publication Data
978-1-4758-6756-5 (cloth)
978-1-4758-6757-2 (paperback)
978-1-4758-6758-9 (electronic)

Contents

FOREWORD

S. Kent Butler, Ph.D., NCC, NCSC

LOOKING AT THE UNSPOKEN! SPEAKING THE TRUTH! WATCHING OUT for a people! Ensuring that reality is checked! *Overlooked: Counselor Insights for the Unspoken Issues in Black American Life* is thirteen phenomenal chapters that provide counselors, helping professionals, and laypeople with an understanding of what it takes to ensure that service providers consistently see and hear the lived realities of Black people! I am impressed with each part of this book, as it provides a rich narrative that supports helping professionals in effectively integrating these unspoken issues into their therapeutic relationships.

Overlooked Identity Issues provides the first stepping stone into understanding a people. There were three words in chapter 1 that struck me. They were "led to believe." I had to sit and honestly ponder the statement that included these words. Their inclusion was, in its own way, profound and exceptionally real. They were eye-opening and incredibly telling. They reminded me of America. They reminded me that in very tangible ways, we have all been led, led astray, led to believe, led . . . maybe . . . to embrace a lot of wrong and hurtful things. Led to inexplicitly cause harm and, in some cases, irrevocable damage.

Often in counseling we look past the client, finding every occasion to talk over and not see the person right in front of us. What is worse is to make flawed assumptions or live with unfounded fear and trepidation. We do this essentially because we do not possess the ability or understanding to meaningfully communicate with Black clients. Many counselors have been dupped to believe that they cannot ever really understand racialized realties because of their own lived realities.

From birth we learn messages that perpetuate our inability to just be our true, wonderfully beautiful, and often imperfect selves. We learn to be afraid of one another or to think we just "know" the truth about someone we have no clue about. We, through inaccurate assumptions, presume to know what others are thinking, going to do, going to say, and it is all because we have never really learned how to just sit and honestly talk with people different from ourselves.

We are in luck because **Overlooked Historical Factors** gives us the language and the necessary tools to have authentic conversations. It helps readers envision how marginalized and oppressed people experience the weight—the intolerance, discrimination, racism, prejudice, exclusion, and emotional toils—of the world. We are told those burdens only existed in the past. We know the truth though. Black individuals endured these historical, horrific experiences throughout the years and unfortunately remain impacted by them in the here-and-now.

Overlooked Clinical Bias opens the readers' eyes to colors they may have never seen before. Maybe we need a new language. Maybe we desperately need a new way of interaction. Maybe we only needed permission from ourselves to just be. Maybe, in fact, we have been mindlessly in a search to find this oh-so-elusive "maybe." *Overlooked: Counselor Insights for the Unspoken Issues in Black American Life* is the resource equipped with the capability to help us stop searching. It gives us that language and ability to see what has always been right here in front of us. Each other! Human Beings!

This powerful resource will spark a revolution and open doors for unlearning dangerous past behaviors toward ALL cultures. It challenges what has blindly been incorporated into the fabric of our unhealthy society: the insidious things that got us to this place; the awfully inhumane things that ought not be a part of human nature; the deceptive things that caused us as a society to become deaf, blind, and mute when it comes to learning and knowing about the people around us.

The Black American community needs allies and co-conspirators who see their value and fight for their mental health needs. They need practitioners who go beyond normal textbook learning and see the **Overlooked Losses** of Black people. The Black community needs counselors who will become lifelong learners: diligently digging deeper into the historical factors that impact the overall growth and development of this multifaceted population; finding appropriate strength-based resources that enable them to connect and build genuine relationships in ways that inspire change and self-love; and practicing in ways that empower and encourage clients from a place of "at-promise" and not one erroneously deemed "at-risk" so that **Overlooked Strengths** never ever go unobserved again.

From a Multicultural and Social Justice Counseling Competencies perspective, this book is a godsend that provides licensed counselors, social workers, marriage and family therapists, addiction counselors, psychologists, pastoral counselors, and other providers an opportunity to look internally and dive into some healing self-reflection. It has the potential to help a person challenge themselves, really question the unknown, and consciously scrutinize their own belief systems.

Each chapter proffers a cultural awareness that is responsive and unpretentious with perspectives that are clinically transformative for Black mental health needs. Infused throughout with the tenets of true social justice advocacy, *Overlooked* helps therapists accurately build case conceptualizations. It includes salient case studies and scenarios that proactively support Black people. Most importantly, it assists in constructing treatment plans that are relevant and make a difference in the lives of Black clients.

LaVerne Hanes Collins sees into a forgotten past, to reveal and bring to the forefront a new view on how counselors may have a genuine impact in the lives of the unvoiced. Overlooked no more, faithful and resilient Black Americans are now watched after with evidence from carefully chosen empirical studies and case studies, such that the unspoken has been given voice. This extraordinary volume provides us with a new love language. Counselors should be thrilled and eager to learn about it and the actionable ways to ensure we see the mission and accomplish the intended results with cultural humility.

Dr. S. Kent Butler
Past President and Fellow, American Counseling Association
Fellow, National Association of Diversity Officers in Higher Education
Professor, Counselor Education
Former Chief Equity, Inclusion and Diversity Officer
University of Central Florida

Overlooked

What Are We Missing?

"If you treat all your clients the same way—regardless of their race or ethnicity—you will be seen as a culturally insensitive therapist. You might even be thought of as racist."

When I make this statement, the reactions of my counseling students and supervisees range from incredulous to teary-eyed. And I understand why. It is simply not what they have been led to believe.

They've been taught to see race neutrality as good, and they find safety in that space. After all, race neutrality is much more comfortable than asking, "As a Black woman/man, how are you doing in light of everything that is going on in our society?" While the inquiry feels far too sensitive for some counselors, cultural sensitivity is actually the goal!

Race-neutral counseling protects the clinician; it is a safeguard against their feelings of vulnerability. However, if a counselor does not consider the role of race in accurate diagnosis, the pain in race-based trauma, the need for values-based interventions, and the importance of cultural support systems, then they deny the client's lived realities. A counselor may find it personally safer to avoid hearing the pain of a racialized experience. The client, however, is left to feel unsafe because this oversight leaves their racial experience on the periphery of the therapeutic discourse.

A race-neutral counselor constructs a plan for addressing work-related stress without regard for how the client is affected by a history of cross-cultural betrayal and justified mistrust that is now woven into the fabric of every interaction.

Race neutrality is a form of ethnocentric thought. From their own ethnocentric lens—presumed to have universal relevance—the counselor treats everyone the same. Not *equitably*, but *the same*. Race-neutral counseling attempts to apply the same explanations and problem conceptualizations to all people. It assumes that what is good for one is also good for another.

To live in the United States is to live in a racialized social system. Yet, counseling students generally get only a cursory look at the issues of racism, ethnicism, and various other -isms. Counselors then enter the professional workforce with universalized tools and expectations for assessment, diagnosis, and treatment interventions with minimal consideration for the nuances of racialized experiences. As a result, counselors can easily overlook some of the most salient factors in a client's lived reality.

This book addresses contemporary concerns for professional counselors in a world where marginalized, racialized, and ethnicized clients are managing high levels of stress, trauma, anxiety, and depression, while simultaneously presenting in counseling with amazing resilience, faith, tenacity, and a strong sense of community. Against this backdrop, it is imperative for counselors to understand their clients' stressors and emerging concerns, but many of these issues remain hidden in the background of the client–counselor conversation.

I wrote this book to lift critical issues out of the shadows—to raise the level of counselors' awareness by uncovering overlooked identity issues, overlooked historical factors, overlooked clinical bias, overlooked losses, and overlooked strengths for Black Americans. Professional counselors and other behavioral health care providers who are effectively engaged in cross-cultural counseling in today's America must be highly aware of the need for cultural humility and race consciousness. Considering the racially charged events of the past decade and ongoing debates about critical race theory, many counselors feel inadequate to address even the most common problems through a multicultural lens.

As a consultant, I see this when I am invited into counseling organizations to provide training or facilitation on multicultural counseling and clinical engagement. I see therapists who fear they will do harm or say the wrong thing. They have concerns about how their own perspectives on race may cause them to cast judgment on the narratives of minoritized people. They recognize ways in which they have mistakenly homogenized their treatment interventions to a one-size-fits-all-races approach without regard for the lived realities of diverse populations.

My audiences are counselors who are aware they have blind spots and are often anxious or tense about missing key factors that their education did not address. This is particularly true of veteran counselors whose educational programs from many years ago did not delve deeply into multicultural issues. Some of those veteran counselors are tenured professors, clinical supervisors, and private-practice clinicians who are concerned about their ability to effectively honor diversity in a multicultural world that requires more from them than their monocultural training prepared them for.

Many providers fear being perceived as racist because of a verbal misstep. Many are afraid they will cause a race rupture that permanently drives a client away. Most fear they will simply overlook something important in a Black client's life.

This book highlights those elements of the Black narrative that are often unseen outside of their communities. It is a book that invites thought about demographic and social factors that other clients do not have to think about. Each chapter brings to light cultural realities that affect Black clients' mental health, help-seeking behavior, perceptions, and expectations. Most importantly, this book aids in the therapist's case conceptualization and thereby can assist in effective treatment planning. Each chapter offers a clinically transformative and culturally informed perspective on Black mental health needs and social justice advocacy for licensed counselors, social workers, marriage and family therapists, addiction counselors, psychologists, pastoral counselors, and other providers.

PART I

OVERLOOKED IDENTITY ISSUES

Naming Rights and Representations

I just took a DNA test. Turns out I'm 100% confused, and that's just about the only thing I know for sure in terms of my identity. Oftentimes, I wish that being confident as a Black woman were enough, or that I was complacent with the idea of just being Black, even though Black (the "color" of my skin) kind of, sort of, completely erases and simplifies what my people and I really are.

At one point, only knowing that my grandparents on both my mother's and father's side were from the South and migrated to the North sufficed. The bare minimum sustained me until I began to meet and converse with people more and more unlike myself: non-Black Americans who could, without hesitation, share and be proud of the country their family originally came from, and who also still practice original traditions. Their traditions had yet to be seized by America and warped until they can no longer belong to just them. Their rituals were still authentic and not yet stigmatized.

And I suppose that was another reason I decided to ship off a glob of my spit to the federal government, where they'll probably save it and later do what they did to Henrietta Lacks. I did it because of what little I knew about myself, what little I owned: the music I listened to, the hairstyles I wore, the Ebonics I spoke. Every little tangible thing that I had was constantly being borrowed but never returned and, quite honestly, ruined.

I was frustrated with trying to search high and low for new things that would make me feel whole. There aren't many scraps of Black culture left to pick from, which is why Black people are constantly creating something new to call our own. While many were and still are okay with redefining themselves, because—trust me—it's a lot easier to do that than all this damn research. It wasn't okay with me. Not anymore, at least. I needed to know who I was at the core./ what I was born from and what I will die as.

In 2017, I begged my mother to buy a DNA kit for my birthday. There were several DNA commercials that played rather frequently at the time, reminding me that knowing was easily accessible. But after getting the results back, I learned that knowing was only accessible if you had more money to dig deeper. What I managed to obtain gave me some gratification while simultaneously shocking me.

I then wondered just how much more I actually needed to know, or better yet, how much of it could I stomach. Apparently, one of my great- or great-great-grandparents is 100% Nigerian and they were born somewhere between 1840 and 1900. Cool. Based off the timeline, that could easily be my granny's mother or her grandmother.

On the opposite end of the spectrum, another one of my great- or great-great-grandparents was 100% British and Irish, again born between 1840 and 1900. I later found out from having a conversation with my father that the 25% European portion of my composition may have come from my great-great- or third-great-grandfather. Apparently, that's only one Google search away too.

The results left many holes. Another ancestor of mine, born between 1780 and 1870, was 100% Ghanaian, Liberian, and Sierra Leonean. The findings traced back a total of eight generations, tossing me into different regions all over western and central Africa, but giving nothing about the exact ethnic groups in these African nations, or better yet, which one out of the 250+ that exist.

Was it Fulani, Yoruba, Akan, Mende, or maybe Igbo? Nothing about the languages, the religions practiced, or forms of art that these groups of people create. Nothing about the food, the history, and experiences rooted in those areas. Nothing about the names of my ancestors that were packed onto ships, may have jumped overboard, or died from starvation, diseases, or endless melancholy.

I learned nothing of their ages. If they left behind children, husbands, or wives. If they were children, husbands, or wives. Nothing that answered all my questions came out of all those numbers. Just more confusion. I even tried to sit with the idea of, "at least you have something to be confused about now" rather than nothing. But that's just settling, accepting what is given to me, though I'm far from satisfied with it. I think Black people have had enough of that already. I wanted more; we want more.

The 23andMe app even noted that much can't be found due to the "disproportionate impact of the Atlantic slave trade," which is just great because outside this app I doubt that I would find more on my own either, due to the "disproportionate impact of the Atlantic slave trade."

Many times, I wondered, as I still do now, where do I go from here? I was in that box now, merely moving forward but hitting a corner every few seconds. I was being turned back around and going over the same patterns and information I already knew. Nothing new appeared, no new results, no reparations, nothing. This was no game of Monopoly. I wish it were.

The only living elder I knew at the time that might have had some info was my granny, but she also had dementia and could barely tell who we were some days, let alone where her antecedents were from. Not even the family reunion booklets we collected every two years could delve past the American end of our lineage.

I then wondered, should I have just been grateful for that too? Be grateful that I'm able to at least trace back the racism that was cast upon my grandparents in the South, that it allegedly ended and "helped" us find modest lives in Chicago? I no longer knew how to feel, what to think, what to identify as. So, I stuck to the less-than-defining "Black" assigned to me.[1]

—Porsha Michelle Stennis

There Is No Telling Who I Am

If I were a client in your office today, the narrative you would hear from the deepest part of *my* soul would sound much like the one you just read. I, too, was extremely excited when I sent my tube of spit to the lab for DNA testing. A few weeks later, I, too, was just as confused as I was excited.

I have taken a dozen or so trips to African nations, and when I read my DNA results, those surreal Motherland experiences came vividly whirling back to my mind! I recalled standing in the dungeons of castle-like forts on the Ghanaian coast of the Atlantic Ocean with family members and friends. We stood where shackled Africans were held, awaiting the next slave cargo ship with no way to comprehend what was about to happen to them.

If I was a client in your office today, I'd want to tell you about the stale stench that still remains in those unventilated dungeons, after all these years, and the horror stories of people dying in the utterly inhumane underground holding spaces that preceded the equally inhumane ship's hold. I'd want to tell you how close I felt to my ancestors every single time I stood in those dungeons. Whoever those African ancestors were, the DNA kit couldn't tell me.

I have been fortunate to visit four of the fifty-four sub-Saharan countries on the continent of Africa. Those countries represent citizenship for their inhabitants, but not tribal lineage. From the late 1800s through the mid-1900s, European nations colonized African regions and created political boundaries to recognize their rule of law over geographic areas. Those colonized areas later became independent nations and thereby created nationalities. However, pre-colonial Africa, or the Africa of the Atlantic Slave Trade, was known for over eight hundred distinct ethnic regions.[2] In other words, while ancestral research may identify a person as having a regional heritage in Nigeria, Liberia, or some other nation, this does not identify the native heritage a slave would have known. Clans and tribes existed at that time; nationalities did not.

If I were a client in your office today, I would also want to tell you how I have been intrigued and made envious by the fact that Africans in major metropolitan areas generally know their ancestral tribe and clan just as well as people who live a quieter life in a rural village with traditional chiefs, elders, and tribal practices. I wish my ancestors could have held onto their native language and their identity without the threat of death. I have learned that the multilingual nation of Ghana, smaller than the state of Michigan in square miles,[3] has more than seventy ethnic groups, each with its own distinct cultural traditions and language: Ewe, Ga, Akan, and others. Today, they know their nationality is merely a geographic assignment. So when an ancestry test identifies an African American like me as 8 percent Ghanaian, it basically assigned me to yet another European category of identification, not to my ancestral clan, tribe, heritage, or culture. So, there is no telling who I am. And I would want to tell you that, too, if I were your client.

In many ways and through many portals, African Americans are reaching for self-identification that predates the horrors of the Transatlantic Slave Trade. This desire has opened the door for DNA test kits marketed specifically to African Americans; and those kits are grow-ing in popularity. Increasingly, advertisements appeal to the desire to have specific ancestral information at the *tribal* level. The thirst for an understandable identity that predates slavery is unquenchable. African American people are investing in the opportunity to know and own a heritage undefined and undefiled by European influence and domination, reclaiming their privilege to self-describe.

What does it mean to stick to the less-than-defining "Black" assigned to people of African descent? Labels, names, tags, and ethnonyms carry weight and meaning. They are either empowering or disempowering. They can be used for identifying or de-identifying. They may serve to validate or invalidate. When a client interacts with a clinician, that client wants to be identified, empowered, and validated. They want to feel seen and respected inside and outside.

When we think about racial identity for members of America's Black communities, it is easy to see skin color and abort any further exploration of self-identification. What does a client *feel* when they identify as Black or African American or Afro-Caribbean? What does it *mean* to them? What are they consciously aware of in their self-identification, and what memories, thoughts, and wounds sit *outside* of their conscious awareness?

Lost Historical Grounding

History shows people where they came from and grounds people in their roots. People develop a sense of kinship and a greater understanding of their ancestors by studying history. Studying the roots and embracing both the past and present-day components of a culture can reveal why members of that culture do certain things and how the past has impacted the present.

Counselors working with African American clients must be careful not to minimize the grief of lost ancestral history. Unlike Europeans who arrived through immigration ports like Ellis Island, African slaves name-lessly entered through other ports and were placed on human auction blocks. Slaves are rarely found in standard genealogical databases prior to 1870, which was the first census year after the Civil War. In fact, from 1619 to 1870, slaves were not considered to be people, but property, and slaveholders counted their slaves primarily for taxation purposes. Even into the early twentieth century, African American births were typically not recorded with birth certificates.

A limited number of slave ship manifests are held in national archives or historical collections. Those documents provided head counts, but trackable leads are a rare find. For the purpose of sale, slavers assigned English given names to each enslaved African. Figure 1.1 is a slave auction announcement from 1858 in New Orleans. This broadside (poster, as we call it today) lists the assigned first name, approximate age, and skills of each person being sold.

Slaves used the last names of the slaveholders on whose property they worked. As a result, African American family names are commonly British surnames. Here are the twenty-five most common surnames in Britain, presented in order of prevalence: Smith, Jones, Williams, Taylor, Davies, Brown, Wilson, Evans, Thomas, Johnson, Roberts, Walker, Wright, Robinson, Thompson, White, Hughes, Edwards, Green, Lewis, Wood, Harris, Martin, Jackson, and Clarke.[4] Compare that list to the twenty-five most common Black/African American surnames in America. In order of prevalence, they are: Williams, Johnson, Smith, Jones, Brown, Jackson, Davis, Thomas, Harris, Robinson, Taylor, Wilson, Moore, White, Lewis, Walker, Green, Thompson, Washington, Anderson, Scott, Carter, Wright, Hill, and Allen.[5] The two lists have about 70 percent congruity.

For all these reasons, detailed genealogy research is complicated and often unfruitful for African Americans. The lost history creates an identity void that counselors should be willing to acknowledge.

WHO DO "YOU-THEY-WE" SAY I AM?

The United States, like many other nations, operates with a human hierarchical structure that assigns assumptions and values to physical features. So when we mention any person by race or ethnicity, there are centuries of bias underneath that label.[6] The historically inequitable treatment of Black people in America has been marked by degrading, demeaning, and contemptuous name-calling. That context adds interracial and intra-racial sensitivity to the self-identity question.

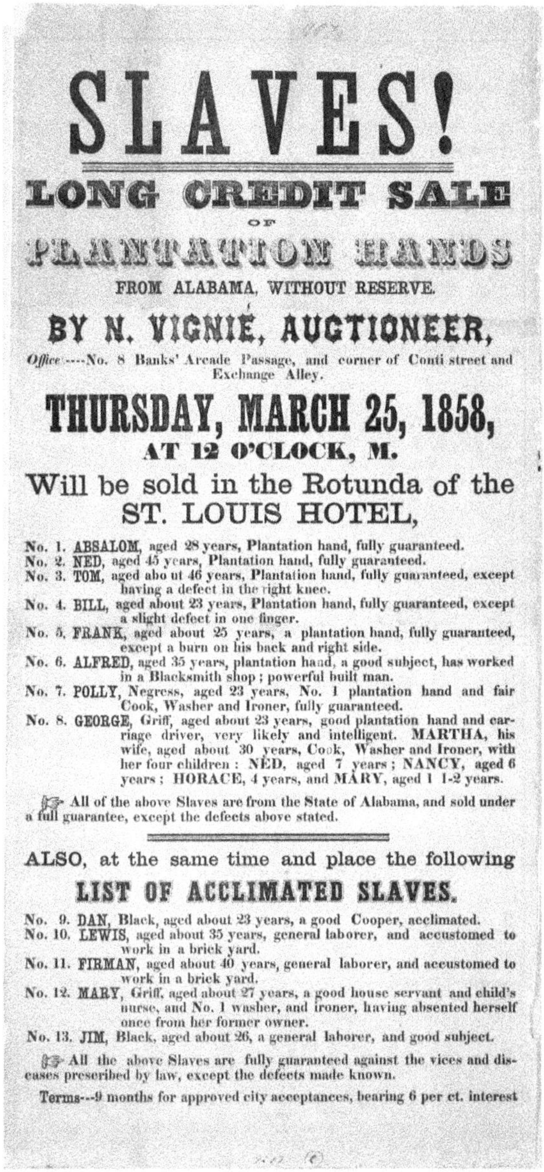

SLAVES!

LONG CREDIT SALE

OF

PLANTATION HANDS

FROM ALABAMA, WITHOUT RESERVE.

BY N. VIGNIÉ, AUCTIONEER,

Office ----No. 8 Banks' Arcade Passage, and corner of Conti street and Exchange Alley.

THURSDAY, MARCH 25, 1858,

AT 12 O'CLOCK, M.

Will be sold in the Rotunda of the ST. LOUIS HOTEL,

No. 1. ABSALOM, aged 28 years, Plantation hand, fully guaranteed.

No. 2. NED, aged 45 years, Plantation hand, fully guaranteed.

No. 3. TOM, aged about 46 years, Plantation hand, fully guaranteed, except having a defect in the right knee.

No. 4. BILL, aged about 23 years, Plantation hand, fully guaranteed, except a slight defect in one finger.

No. 5. FRANK, aged about 25 years, a plantation hand, fully guaranteed, except a burn on his back and right side.

No. 6. ALFRED, aged 35 years, plantation hand, a good subject, has worked in a Blacksmith shop ; powerful built man.

No. 7. POLLY, Negress, aged 23 years, No. 1 plantation hand and fair Cook, Washer and Ironer, fully guaranteed.

No. 8. GEORGE, Griff, aged about 23 years, good plantation hand and carriage driver, very likely and intelligent. MARTHA, his wife, aged about 30 years, Cook, Washer and Ironer, with her four children : NED, aged 7 years ; NANCY, aged 6 years ; HORACE, 4 years, and MARY, aged 1 1-2 years.

☞ All of the above Slaves are from the State of Alabama, and sold under a full guarantee, except the defects above stated.

ALSO, at the same time and place the following

LIST OF ACCLIMATED SLAVES.

No. 9. DAN, Black, aged about 23 years, a good Cooper, acclimated.

No. 10. LEWIS, aged about 35 years, general laborer, and accustomed to work in a brick yard.

No. 11. FIRMAN, aged about 40 years, general laborer, and accustomed to work in a brick yard.

No. 12. MARY, Griff, aged about 27 years, a good house servant and child's nurse, and No. 1 washer, and ironer, having absented herself once from her former owner.

No. 13. JIM, Black, aged about 26, a general laborer, and good subject.

☞ All the above Slaves are fully guaranteed against the vices and diseases prescribed by law, except the defects made known.

Terms---9 months for approved city acceptances, bearing 6 per ct. interest

Figure 1.1. Auction announcement for the sale of 18 enslaved persons from Alabama on March 25, 1858, in New Orleans, Louisiana.

SOURCE: COLLECTION OF THE SMITHSONIAN NATIONAL MUSEUM OF AFRICAN AMERICAN HISTORY AND CULTURE, WASHINGTON, DC. OBJECT NUMBER 2011.155.305 (PUBLIC DOMAIN).

Racism is verbally and psychologically violent. So, even more salient than the issue of "how do we identify ourselves?" and "how do we prefer others to describe us?" is the painful fact that these questions of collective identity are an issue to be pondered at all. A thin line has existed between the naming and name-calling of Black Americans. Until the 1970s, African Americans were forced to accept both the name-calling and the assigned naming of their race while resigning themselves to their voicelessness in those decisions.

The descendants of African slavery in America have been racially renamed just about every decade or two since the early 1900s. That is the subjective nature of social identities. The racial designations have evolved and shifted, setting expectations, social location, and norms that affect every dimension of life.

Let us trace the history of racial identity designations for people of African descent in America: Darkies, Negroes, and Aethiops, (1600s–late 1800s); Colored people (1900–1940s); Negro race (1950s–1960s); Blacks (1970s–1980s); Afro-American /African American (1980s–1990's); Black, again (2000); People of Color (2010); and more recently Black, Indigenous, and People of Color abbreviated as BIPOC (2019–present). The ascribed identity language for your generation of Black determined how you would be treated by others and what was expected of you, especially in southern states. Of course, those decades are not absolute, but they are meant to represent approximate time periods and illustrate the slow trend toward more respectful racial designations, as people of African descent searched to own a meaningful, representative, social identity in America, beyond "the N-word."

"The N-word"—a familiar euphemistic expression for the word "nigger," is a carryover from slavery and conveys the utmost disrespect and contempt. Use this euphemism and everyone knows exactly what it means. The substitutionary use of "N-word," as a verbal evasion, evolved because people needed a politically correct substitute that would save them from experiencing social consequences when quoting *someone else's* use of the word "nigger" in racially diverse company.[7] In all this, the paradox is that labels are powerful markers of social identity, but one's self-identity is psychologically more powerful than a label.

The Call for a Collective Identity with Cultural Integrity

The Reverend Jesse Jackson is credited with publicly introducing the campaign advocating for the use of "African American" in place of the term "Black" in December 1988. "Just as we were called Colored, but were not that, and then Negro, but not that, to be called Black is just as baseless," Jackson said, following a meeting with other national representatives of Black/African American organizations. "To be called African Americans has cultural integrity," he said. "It puts us in our proper historical context. Every ethnic group in this country has a reference to some land base, some historical cultural base. African Americans have hit that level of cultural maturity." Jackson added, "There are Armenian Americans and Jewish Americans and Arab Americans and Italian Americans, and with a degree of accepted and reasonable pride, they connect their heritage to their mother country and where they are now."[8]

This was a pivotal moment! African Americans determined how they would be identified within their race and by others, telling the world how to respect the heritage of slavery's descendants. But there were also pivotal questions. At that time, I personally wondered if the use of "African American" would really bring about a greater sense of pride and consciousness for people of African descent in America? Would it catch on interracially? Intra-racially? Intergenerationally? Or was "African American" just a matter of semantics with no sociopolitical muscle? Would the world finally recognize American-born people of African descent as a distinct and respected ethnic group, equal to other groups?

Moreover, was this new term weaker than the strength asserted in the "Black Power" and "Black Is Beautiful" slogans of the 1960s and 1970s? In retrospect, the declarations that first ascribed beauty and power to Blackness were necessary precursors for the day when an entire race of people would be invited by their national leaders to reject the dominant culture's labels and exercise their right to choose—and then use—their own identifier.

For many people, it really is just a matter of semantics. Black and African American are often used interchangeably in writing and conversation. They are regularly used to broadly classify *all* people of African descent living in the United States. However, Black people are not literally black, and White people are not literally white—many people called White have darker skin tones than someone who is called Black. As such, the color terms are poor metonyms for either group, but it's what we have.

Counselors must recognize each person's preferences; every descendant of slavery does not self-identify as African American. It is a matter of nativity, self-perception, and representation. Some believe it is disingenuous to identify as "African American," saying, "I don't know anything about what it means to be from Africa. It doesn't feel like it's right for me to claim that I'm *African* American. I identify as Black." This perspective holds that true transnationalism requires a physical or psychological connection to two identities. In the absence of knowing one's genealogical or ancestral history on the continent of Africa, a dual identifier like African American feels illegitimate. Their African friends in the United States may even suggest that the term "African American" is not appropriate for someone who has no direct knowledge of Africa.

Others say, "Why would you call yourself Black? Black is the color used to represent death and evil things. I am an African American. I am not a color, and I am especially not a color that represents all things demonized." This debate takes place between family members, friends, coworkers, and other acquaintances, often with great conviction. It is an intra-racial struggle resulting from the historical assault on the identity of people of African descent in America.

People of Afro-Caribbean descent, preferring to use their island heritage to self-identify, may say, "I'm not African American; my people are from Jamaica, or Haiti, or Barbados, and I am a Jamaican, Haitian, or Bajan (Barbadian)." Other individuals may prefer to recognize both their specific ancestral ethnicity and their American citizenship, as with Jamaican Americans or Haitian Americans.

African immigrants also have a different sense of identity. Culturally sensitive counselors must ensure that African immigrants are seen and heard for who they are. It is most appropriate to use specific national references such as Kenyan, Nigerian, Ghanaian, etc., if the specific tribe or ethnic group is unknown. Second-generation African descendants may prefer to recognize both their ancestral ethnicity and their American citizenship, as with Nigerian Americans or Ghanaian Americans.

By observation, African American, Afro-Caribbean, and African immigrants are often not distinguishable. So, we broadly define "Black" as a person having genealogical origins in any of the Black racial groups of Africa. This includes American-born, Caribbean-born, and people born in Sub-Saharan Africa. Some identify as Black alone while others identify as Black in combination with one or more other race or ethnic groups (e.g., Black and White, Black and Hispanic, or Black and Asian). It was not until 2020 that the US Census Bureau changed how it asked Black people to designate their race, with expanded options such as African American, Jamaican, Haitian, Nigerian, Ethiopian, Ghanaian, South African, Barbadian, Kenyan, Liberian, and Bahamian.

Cultural Repression

First-generation enslaved Africans lived with the traumatic shock of slavery in a strange land with cruel treatment. Their cultural representations and practices were forbidden in America, but they still had their memories of life in Africa. The slaveholders disallowed all aspects of culture—tribal languages, names, music, dances, and other cultural forms of expression—as a means of preventing any secret communication of uprisings or escape plans. As a result, first-generation slaves were most significantly impacted by the cultural loss.

Subsequent generations of slaves were impacted differently. Beginning with second-generation slaves, there was no knowledge of a different way of life in Africa. At best, they may have heard memories shared secretly by their parents, but the risk of sharing such stories was grave. With no connection to their homeland, they were left to create new communities and identities.

The sociological term for living with the dual realities of two cultures is "hybrid identity." Voluntary immigrants can bring their culture of origin and intersect it with their host culture. When this hybrid identity is created, the identities are not separately assimilated or transformed; rather, aspects of the two cultures are merged into the formation of a new hybrid culture. Unlike voluntary immigrants, African Americans have not had the privilege of developing this hybrid identity in America. Slaves in colonial America were given no freedom to be African in culture, either in part or in whole, and no rights to the freedoms America touted. In his book, *The Souls of Black Folk*, W. E. B. Du Bois said that there is no merging, only two types of consciousness at war within one life:

> It is a peculiar sensation, this double consciousness, this sense of always looking at oneself through the eyes of others, of measuring one's soul by the tape of a world that looks on in amused contempt and pity. One ever feels his two-ness,—an American, a Negro; two souls, two thoughts, two unreconciled strivings; two warring ideals in one dark body, whose dogged strength alone keeps it from being torn asunder.[9]

With a hybrid identity, two cultures interact within the individual person such that each cultural perspective informs and influences the other and creates a new identity that is distinct within each context. People can experience themselves and their identities through both cultural lenses. This was not afforded to slaves and their descendants—human beings whose primary identity was perpetually devalued.

It is the counselor's responsibility to honor the client's preferences for racial/ethnic self-identification in the counseling relationship. It is important for each person to self-identify in ways that are most meaningful to them. Table 1.1 provides a summary view of nomenclature used for people of African descent. Take note of the meanings, acceptability, limitations, and usages of each term.

RACE AS MASTER STATUS

In sociology, "master status" is a term denoting the social status that is most defining for an individual. Everett Hughes coined this term, with special reference to race as the primary identifier for racialized people. People generally do not have just one status, but a "status set" consisting of all the statuses they hold simultaneously. A person can have "ascribed status," an involuntary status into which they are born. They may also have "achieved status," into which they enter voluntarily by way of their accomplishments. Common statuses are those of age, gender assignment, race or ethnicity, sexual orientation, ability, educational attainment, religion or spirituality, or profession.[10] Some of those are achieved, and others are ascribed.

For people of African descent in America, race is the status most likely to outweigh the other characteristics in their status set. In other words, a Black person is most known for being Black. They will be described in conversations as a Black doctor, a Black pastor, a Black teacher, or a Black attorney, while Whites are simply described as a doctor, a pastor, a teacher, or an attorney. A Black person might *want* their professional achievement to be their master status, but in the American system, race is the master status for a Black person no matter what they have *achieved*. The meaning an African American person gives to this master status—what it means to be Black in America—will either propel them (if that meaning is positive) or stall them (if it is negative). This makes racial and ethnic identity critical for Black Americans.

> A Black person might *want* their professional achievement to be their master status, but in the American system, race is the master status for a Black person no matter what they have *achieved*.

Mental health providers might overlook the pain of a Black person's experience of being known more for their race than their achievements. Counselors might underestimate the struggle born out of the client's ascribed master status. This mistake is evident in statements like "I can't imagine you've been held back by racism because you've accomplished so much in your lifetime." Clinicians would do well to recognize that a Black person may become weary of a social position defined by their race.

RACIAL AND ETHNIC IDENTITY AND MEANING-MAKING

Identity development involves knowing and understanding oneself within the context of societal norms and cultural demands.[11] Meaning-making, as a coping model, involves understanding one's own experiences in a way that helps make sense of life events. Thus, racial and ethnic identity development and meaning-making are inextricably intertwined in Black American life.

TABLE 1.1. Historical and Current Terms for Afrocentric Identities

Term	Guidelines for Use
African	A native or inhabitant of the continent of Africa. Typically, this is reserved for a person of African ancestry who is from a specific geographical region or people originating from Sub-Saharan Africa. This term may also be used as a prefix or descriptor of origin for specific groups living in another country (e.g., African American, African Caribbean, African Canadian). Culturally respectful users of this term will consider that Africa is a continent with heterogeneous populations and nations. While the word "African" may be used generally, the reference to a specific national origin is preferred when it is known (e.g., Liberian, Rwandan, or Kenyan) to avoid over-generalizing or treating Africa as a cultural monolith.
African American	A Black citizen of the United States with African ancestry or a mix of African with European American ancestry; usually a descendent of slavery. This term was introduced by national Black leaders in 1988 to be used in place of the term "Black." The term was chosen because it acknowledges both the genealogical heritage of Africa and also present citizenship in the United States of America. Culturally respectful usage avoids applying this term as a catch-all for broader heterogeneous groups. Not all "Blacks" in the U.S. are African American. The term may also be used as a name for the *ethnicity* and *culture* of Black descendants of slavery in the United States.
Afro-Caribbean	A person of African ancestry who is a native of a wide range of islands and cultures in the Caribbean region. The term may also be used as a name for the culture or for the geographic region itself. Culturally respectful usage avoids applying this term as a catch-all if individuals prefer to recognize both their specific ancestral ethnicity and their American citizenship (e.g., Jamaican American, Haitian American).
Black	A member of a racial group with African or Caribbean ancestry. The term allows for a collective identity for people of African descent but may also hide the heterogeneity and cultures of diverse people by combining them under an umbrella category. While this term is preferred by some, it is rejected by others. In general, this is a term acceptable for culturally respectful inclusion of all people of African ancestry regardless of ethnicity or nationality.

Term	Guidelines for Use
Black, Indigenous and People of Color	This collective term, commonly abbreviated as "BIPOC," is used to broadly describe populations who have a history of systemic marginalization in the United States because of their racial, ethnic, or cultural identity. This marginalization includes historical, intergenerational and race-based trauma. "Black" generally describes people of African or Caribbean descent. "Indigenous" describes native inhabitants of North America, including Alaska. People of Color is a broad term for anyone who is not White and may include Latinx, Asians, Pacific Islanders, and others. This term attempts to shift away from the use of the word "minority." Culturally respectful usage does not use the term as a non-White melting pot. Instead, the term is intended to acknowledge that although not all people of color have the same experiences with racist structures and discrimination, they all have been harmed by those structures.
Colored	This term was once used to describe any person belonging to a racial group not categorized as White, but especially for a person of African descent or a person of mixed race. The term is associated with slavery and Jim Crow–era segregation and was commonly used and accepted until the Civil Rights Movement. Today, this term is generally offensive and should always be avoided.
Negro	This is another term that was assigned to people of African descent and associated with slavery and Jim Crow segregation. It was commonly used and accepted until the 1960s. The term was associated with the word "nigger" (a highly disrespectful insult). Today, the word Negro is generally offensive and should be avoided because of its highly derogatory connotation. The category "Black, African American, or Negro" was last used in the 2000 census, based on research that showed there was an older cohort of African Americans who still often self-identified as "Negro." It was not an option on the 2010 census form.
People of Color	This is a broad term for anyone who is not White. It is used to describe anyone who has been adversely affected by racism, discrimination, or White supremacy. The term is still acceptable, but is increasingly being considered outdated. Its limitation is that it presents all racialized and ethnicized people as homogenous, and does not provide for the distinction of unique experiences such as Native invisibility, anti-Blackness, and stereotypes against Hispanic/Latinx groups. "People of Color" is often seen as the person-first version of "Colored people," meaning that the word "people" precedes rather than follows the label of Colored.

NOTE: DICTIONARY-DERIVED MEANINGS COME MAINLY FROM THE *AMERICAN HERITAGE DICTIONARY OF THE ENGLISH LANGUAGE* HTTPS://WWW .AHDICTIONARY.COM/ AND FROM THE *MERRIAM-WEBSTER DICTIONARY* HTTPS://WWW.MERRIAM-WEBSTER.COM/DICTIONARY/.

It is an evolution of sorts, based on the conclusions a Black person reaches when they look at the world and psychologically position themselves in it. Many socialization questions arise: How does the world perceive me? What do I believe about how others perceive me? Do I believe the world values my personhood as a member of the Black community? Am I perceived as a threat or an asset? And for each answer, where does that perception evolve from? People who face more racial discrimination tend to give more importance to the racial parts of their identities.[12] So, when it comes to carrying the burden of racial discrimination, a positive cultural identity is an important buffer[13] that Black people must fight to retain for themselves and their descendants in a society that has used their identity against them.

Managing the emotional and psychological weight of anti-Black bias and discrimination using one's master status requires a strong sense of self and a positive sense of community. These are derived from a combination of ethnic identity, racial identity, racial regard, and racial centrality. Such are the quintessential elements that give meaning to a person's Black identity.

Ethnic and Racial Identity

Ethnic identification includes a sense of belonging to a group related by heritage, traditions, values, and languages.[14] This is distinct from racial identity, which is primarily a function of, and response to, being categorized by racism.[15] Nonetheless, the significance and meaning that African Americans place on their race has a powerful impact on their development and life experience.[16] Racial identification provides a sense of collective association, based on the perception of shared racial heritage with a specific group.[17]

Studies show that racial identity is an important psychosocial resource with implications for African Americans' health.[18] Research suggests that African American female college students with a stronger racial identity will show signs of better mental health than their peers who are in an earlier stage of racial identity development.[19] Because those peers were in the pre-encounter stage or had a less developed racial identity, they had constructed a pro-White and anti-Black worldview. A greater awareness of race reflects a healthier response to a social environment that is frequently ambiguous or hostile in terms of racial discrimination.[20]

Racial Regard

Researchers have also given attention to racial regard, which is how someone feels about being in a group, or about broader ideas exploring racial/ethnic identity. Racial regard comes from a model of collective self-esteem developed by Luhtanen and Crocker in 1992.[21] The concept of racial regard is often recognized as a part of racial/ethnic meaning-making. Racial regard consists of positive feelings and pride toward one's racial/ethnic group and is a strong predictor of self-esteem among African American, Latino, and White adolescents.[22]

Racial Centrality

Lastly, the concept of racial centrality is also increasingly recognized as an important dimension of racial and ethnic identity. Racial centrality refers to a normative self-definition in terms of race or the significance of a person's Black identity to their sense of self.[23] Studies show that a more central Black identity is associated with greater psychological well-being and reduces the detrimental effects of prejudicial discrimination on health.[24] Research with African American teens has shown that racial regard will only lead to positive outcomes if race or ethnicity is a central part of a person's identity.[25]

Counselors should listen for indications of strong racial identity, racial regard, and racial centrality. To miss signs of racial meaning-making may mean the omission of therapeutic content that could strengthen the client's overall wellbeing.

THE SALIENCE OF IDENTITY DISCUSSIONS

What it means to be Black in America is complex and multifaceted, affecting every area of life. Clinicians must not dismiss the salience of identity discussions with clients and must be prepared to effectively broach issues of culture. Some providers may worry that bringing these sensitive issues to the foreground will sound racist: "If I introduce the topic of discrimination as one of their stressors, I am afraid the client will think I only see their skin color. I also don't want them to think I view them as weak."

But the research tells a different story: White counselors who address racial and cultural factors are deemed to be more credible than those who ignore those factors.[26] When a client of color experiences race, ethnicity, and culture as important identity dimensions, but perceives their counselor as lacking the capacity to broach those topics, that client will likely disengage from therapy and choose to meet their needs with family or friends who they view as safe.[27] So, let's talk about it. Those are the pages in a client's story that need not be overlooked. They need to be read aloud.

NOTES

1. Porsha Michelle Stennis, "The Black American Identity Quiz," *The Syndrome Mag* (July 20, 2020), https://thesyndromemag.com/the-black-american-identity-quiz.

2. Caitlin Finlayson, "Pre-Colonial, Sub-Saharan Africa," University of Mary Washington, *Social Sci Libre Texts,* August 16, 2020, accessed January 28, 2023, https://socialsci.libretexts.org/Bookshelves/Geography_(Human)/Book%3A_World_Regional_Geography_(Finlayson)/06%3A_Sub-Saharan_Africa/6.02%3A_Pre-Colonial_Sub-Saharan_Africa.

3. "List of African Countries by Area," *Statistics Times*, 2021, https://statisticstimes.com/geography/african-countries-by-area.php; US Census Bureau, "State Area Measurements and Internal Point Coordinates," *Census.gov*, December 16, 2021, https://www.census.gov/geographies/reference-files/2010/geo/state-area.html. The West African nation of Ghana has a total area of 92,098 square miles, while Michigan has a total area of 96,714 square miles.

4. Tom Embury-Dennis, "The 25 Most Common Surnames in Britain—And What They Say about Your Family History," *Independent,* November 18, 2016, https://www.independent.co.uk/news/uk/home-news/the-25-common-surnames-britain-family-history-university-west-england-bristol-uk-a7423196.html.

5. "Most Common Black Last Names in the United States," Name Census, accessed March 31, 2023, https://namecensus.com/last-names/common-black-surnames.

6. Isabel Wilkerson, *Caste: The Origins of Our Discontents* (New York: Random House, 2020), 18.

7. Within the African American community, particularly among adolescent and young adult males, the word "Nigga" may be used jovially, but acceptance is limited to use within their own social circle; "Nigga," *UrbanDictionary.com*, February 2, 2008, https://www.urbandictionary.com/define.php?term=nigga.

8. Associated Press, "Leaders Say Blacks Want to be Called 'African-Americans,'" December 20, 1988, accessed March 31, 2023. https://apnews.com/article/089fc3ab25b86e14deeefae3adb7a5ad.

9. W. E. B. Du Bois, The Souls of Black Folk (Lit2Go Edition, (1903), accessed April 03, 2023, https://etc.usf.edu/lit2go/203/the-souls-of-black-folk/4428/chapter-1-of-our -spiritual-strivings.

10. Everett Cherrington Hughes, "Dilemmas and Contradictions of Status," *American Journal of Sociology* 50, no. 5 (March 1945): 353–59, http://www.jstor.org/stable/2771188.

11. "Identity Development," Psychology.iresearchnet.com, October 9, 2016, accessed March 21, 2023, http://psychology.iresearchnet.com/counseling-psychology/identity -development.

12. Linda Charmaraman and Jennifer M. Grossman, "Importance of Race and Ethnicity: An Exploration of Asian, Black, Latino, and Multiracial Adolescent Identity," *Cultural Diversity & Ethnic Minority Psychology* 16, no. 2 (April 2010): 144–51, https:// doi.org/10.1037/a0018668.

13. Courtney S. Thomas Tobin et al., "Early Life Racial Discrimination, Racial Centrality, and Allostatic Load Among African American Older Adults," *The Gerontologist* 62, no. 5 (June 2022): 721–31, https://doi.org/10.1093/geront/gnab185.

14. Jean S. Phinney and Anthony D. Ong, "Conceptualization and Measurement of Ethnic Identity: Current Status and Future Directions, *Journal of Counseling Psychology* 54, no. 3 (2007): 271–81, https://doi.org/10.1037/0022-0167.54.3.271.

15. Janet E. Helms, "Some Better Practices for Measuring Racial and Ethnic Identity Constructs," *Journal of Counseling Psychology* 54, no. 3 (2007): 235–46, https://doi.org/10 .1037/0022-0167.54.3.235.

16. Cleopatra Howard Caldwell, et al., "Racial Identity, Maternal Support, and Psychological Distress Among African American Adolescents," *Child Development* 73, no. 4 (July–August 2002): 1322–36, https://doi.org/10.1111/1467-8624.00474.

17. David H. Demo and Michael Hughes, "Socialization and Racial Identity among Black Americans," *Social Psychology Quarterly* 53, no. 4 (December 1990): 364–74, https: //doi.org/10.2307/2786741.

18. Caldwell et al., "Racial Identity," 1323; Helena E. Dagadu and C. André Christie-Mizell, "Heart Trouble and Racial Group Identity: Exploring Ethnic Heterogeneity Among Black Americans," *Race and Social Problems* 6, no. 2 (June 2014): 143–60, https://doi.org/10.1007/s12552-013-9109-7.

19. Carlton T. Pyant and Barbara J. Yanico, "Relationship of Racial Identity and Gender-Role Attitudes to Black Women's Psychological Well-Being," *Journal of Counseling Psychology* 38, no. 3 (1991): 315–22, https://doi.org/10.1037/0022-0167.38.3.315.

20. Pyant and Yanico, "Relationship of Racial Identity," 315–22.

21. Riia Luhtanen and Jennifer Crocker, "A Collective Self-Esteem Scale: Self-Evaluation of One's Social Identity," *Personality and Social Psychology Bulletin* 18, no. 3 (June 1992): 302–18, https://doi.org/10.1177/0146167292183006.

22. Jean S. Phinney, Cindy Lou Cantu, and Dawn A. Kurtz, "Ethnic and American Identity as Predictors of Self-Esteem Among African American, Latino, and White Adolescents," *Journal of Youth and Adolescence* 26, no. 2 (April 1997): 165–85, https://doi .org/10.1023/A:1024500514834.

23. Tiffany Yip, Eleanor K. Seaton, and Robert M. Sellers, "African American Racial Identity Across the Lifespan: Identity Status, Identity Content, and Depressive

Symptoms, *Child Development* 77, no. 5 (September–October 2006): 1504–17, https://doi.org/10.1111/j.1467-8624.2006.00950.x.

24. Robert M. Sellers and J. Nicole Shelton, "The Role of Racial Identity in Perceived Racial Discrimination," *Journal of Personality and Social Psychology* 84, no. 5 (May 2003): 1079–92, https://doi.org/10.1037/0022-3514.84.5.1079; Caldwell *et al.*, "Racial Identity," 1322–36.

25. Caldwell et al., "Racial Identity," 1322–36; Tabbye M. Chavous et al., "Gender Matters, Too: The Influences of School Racial Discrimination and Racial Identity on Academic Engagement Outcomes Among African American Adolescents," *Developmental Psychology* 44, no. 3 (May 2008): 637–54, https://doi.org/10.1037/0012-1649.44.3.637.

26. Naijian Zhang and Alan W. Burkard, "Client and Counselor Discussions of Racial and Ethnic Differences in Counseling: An Exploratory Investigation," *Journal of Multicultural Counseling and Development* 36, no. 2 (April 2008): 77–87, https://doi.org/10.1002/j.2161-1912.2008.tb00072.x.

27. Donald B. Pope-Davis et al., "Client Perspectives of Multicultural Counseling Competence, *The Counseling Psychologist* 30, no. 3 (May 2002): 355–93, https://doi.org/10.1177/0011000002303001.

CHAPTER 2

Understanding the Diaspora

More than Black

Who we are as African Americans, as black folks in the diaspora, our cultural destiny, has been shaped by both the enslaved and the free.[1]

—BELL HOOKS

"DIASPORA" IS A WORD MEANING "PEOPLE SETTLED FAR FROM THEIR ancestral homelands."[2] The term is applied when people from one common place are dispersed to other places. In Chapter 1, we introduced some key distinctions. In the United States, there is an African diaspora composed of diverse groups, including African Americans, Afro-Caribbean Islanders, and African nationals from various ethnic cultures and nations in Sub-Saharan Africa. These diasporic groupings represent ethnicities with sociocultural variations based on native birthplace, experiences, and other cultural factors. The sociocultural variations are notable, but not always noticeable. Because of their shared physical traits, the groups can be difficult to distinguish. This phenomenon is known as "invisibility." If counselors mistakenly view people of African descent as an ethnic monolith of African Americans, important sociocultural variations and the related implications for culturally responsive mental health care are overlooked.

DIASPORAN DISTINCTIONS

African diasporans arrived in the United States under a range of circumstances. Some diasporans are descendants of African slaves. Most of slavery's descendants in America now carry varying degrees of mixed ancestry, with the average African American genome being nearly a quarter European.[3] Evidence of this mixed ancestry can be seen in the wide range of skin tones and hair textures among African Americans.

Some people of African descent in America do not identify as African American because their lineage is not connected to early American history. In more recent decades, these diasporans arrived as immigrants from the Caribbean and from African nations. Many came with ample resources and hopes for new opportunities in education or business. Others came as refugees or asylum-seekers, bringing the desire to escape persecution, wars, or natural disasters. Thus, the range of African diasporan experiences in the United States is significantly influenced by the varied circumstances that brought them or their ancestors to this continent. The ways in which those circumstances and ethnic identities inform their expectations and their lived realities is often overlooked.

We have examined how the nomenclature shift from "Black" to "African American" was gradually accepted into American language convention for the descendants of chattel slavery. Yet, the "African American" identifier is easily over-applied. When the term "African American" is used indiscriminately for all "Blacks" and applied solely on the basis of skin color and phenotypic features, a large portion of the African diaspora is mistakenly absorbed into the history of chattel slavery and all that has ensued since then. To do this is to treat phenotypic similarities as the only measure of ethnicity—it is like saying all dark-haired Europeans must be Italian! The reality is that Black cultures in America represent diverse diasporic experiences that translate into ethnic and cultural differences.

While there is significant diversity within the African diaspora, "Black" is still used as the collective term to describe any person of African descent. However, the individual's sociocultural variation is best recognized using specific identifiers such as Jamaican American, African American, Nigerian American, and other nativity acknowledgements.

Nomenclature that recognizes one's native home and also their current land always provides a more accurate cultural and ethnic descriptor.

In different ways, *all* the African diasporan groups in the United States have been subjected to racist attitudes, discriminatory actions, race-based trauma, and inadequate medical and mental health care on the basis of their skin color.[4] How people of these diverse African ethnicities perceive those experiences and build their racial identity has a profound influence on how they navigate their social milieu, their mental health, and their help-seeking patterns.[5] For this reason, it is imperative for counselors not to dismiss distinctions between African American, Afro-Caribbean, and African ethnic experiences in America.

This level of conceptual clarity requires that counselors recognize the interconnections between nativity and cultural influences as essential tools for effectively addressing mental health in our increasingly diverse nation. Scholars point out that even many sociologists have overlooked these sociocultural variations when considering sources of stress and mental health status.[6] To continue to do so is both culturally unresponsive and irresponsible. It is incumbent upon counselors to recognize and honor the ethnic diversity that exists in Black American life.

SLAVERY'S DESCENDANTS

From the mid-1500s through the late 1800s, much of the American labor force was composed of enslaved African men, women, and children. The slaves were traded or captured on the continent of Africa and involuntarily transported in cargo ships to the Americas. The sole purpose of slavery was to provide colonizers with an unpaid labor force for building their wealth. Colonizers unscrupulously displaced the Indigenous people of this continent and built their own versions of the European cultures from which they had come. The United States of America became a nation built on stolen land using stolen labor.

African Americans are the descendants of that stolen labor force. Their forefathers arrived on slave transport ships and were sold or auctioned off to the highest bidder. They were husbands, wives, sons, daughters, sisters, and brothers—but they were classified as property, not as human beings. Among them were kings and queens, chiefs and traditional healers, craftsmen and tradesmen, farmers, hunters and fishermen, cooks and garment-makers, basket weavers, carpenters, musicians, and artists from a culture and civilization misunderstood and devalued by the Europeans.

They were owned and subject to control under chattel slavery, which was a "total institution."[7] Comparable to how a jail oversees its prisoners' daily lives, the total institution of chattel slavery managed every aspect of a slave's existence. Slavery left its victims scarred in ways that are unmistakable. Cruelty, rape, limited freedom, beatings, disrespect for human life, and complete control are some of the aspects of a slave's existence that have left a lasting imprint on their descendants.

Research suggests that many damaging effects of traumatic experiences are retained in the body and can be passed on to subsequent generations.[8] One landmark study found that the stress hormone profiles of Holocaust survivors have been passed down intergenerationally. In that study, the survivors' altered hormone patterns were still evident in their offspring, generations later, in ways that were notably different from their peers. This type of traumatic inheritance can make children more prone to developing post-traumatic stress disorder and contribute to them having a harder time recovering from traumatic experiences.[9]

The descendants of slaves may also be carrying the effects of a significant amount of historical trauma, both experientially and epigenetically, as a result of nearly three hundred years of ancestral slavery, one hundred years of Jim Crow laws throughout parts of the country, and more than fifty additional years of systemic and institutional discrimination after the Jim Crow era. When someone questions why African Americans do not "just get over it" (slavery), they don't realize it is like saying, "Why haven't you fixed your stress hormone profiles yet?" Counselor sensitivity to this little-known fact could change clinical interventions and outcomes for African American clients.

The slave trade was largely responsible for the United States' sizable and growing Black population for centuries,[10] but descendants of slaves are just one group of people of African descent in the United States. As time passed, the African diaspora also grew through voluntary immigration.

IMMIGRANTS

Free and voluntary Black migration to the United States is a relatively new development.[11] Here are a few key findings from the Pew Research Center about Black immigrants. One out of every ten Black people in the United States is an immigrant.[12] Since 1970, the number of Sub-Saharan Africans and Afro-Caribbeans migrating to the United States has surged.[13] Together, these two regions accounted for 88 percent of all foreign-born Black people in the United States in 2019.[14] Roughly 21 percent of the US Black population are immigrants or children of Black immigrants and more than half (58 percent) of those arrived in the United States after 2000.[15] This includes those who identify as Black only, multiracial Black, or Black Hispanic.[16] The US Census Bureau projects that the total foreign-born Black population will more than double by 2060, to 9.5 million.[17] Despite being a sizable and rapidly growing demographic group, Black immigrants to the United States have received disproportionately little attention for their diverse characteristics and mental health.

Approximately 2.1 million immigrants from Sub-Saharan Africa resided in the United States in 2019.[18] Despite research and policy attempts to address health inequities among immigrant communities, African immigrants in the United States remain the least researched immigrant group. They are frequently included with other phenotypically similar groups in the Black category despite having distinct health care requirements and experiences, which makes it challenging to use research data to inform important mental and physical health care targeting their specific needs.[19]

In interviews with a small sample of seven transnational Black women from Antigua, Guyana, Barbados, Grenada, and Trinidad living in Brooklyn, New York, a team of researchers examined how the women perceive race and ethnicity in the United States. Several important points arose in their findings.[20] The interviews revealed that Black immigrants have both a pre- and post-migration understanding of their race. Before migrating, they are part of a Black majority population; after they move, they are part of a racially minoritized population. As a result, Black immigrant clients may experience a kind of duality or uncertainty regarding their racial place in society. These two different stances fluctuate depending on the situation and societal norms. For instance, outside of their own communities, Black immigrants may be seen as African Americans due to their phenotypic expressions such as skin color. They may also be treated in ways that are new to them and face unfamiliar stereotypical expectations.[21]

Whether your ancestors arrived in 1620 on a slave ship, or you arrived in 2020 on a jumbo jet, discrimination awaited anyone with dark skin.

When assumptions are made about an individual's identity and used against them, the individual can feel misunderstood, ashamed, or anxious.[22] This lack of control over how they are regarded by others adds complexity not just to how they think about themselves but also to their clinical presentation. These considerations are easily overlooked in counseling and may need to be broached by the counselor using gentle inquiry and reflective listening as the client presents their narrative. Counseling may need to include conversations that empower Black immigrants as they navigate their conceptions of self and deconstruct the conventional racial misperceptions that society places upon them.[23]

Once Black immigrants have arrived in the United States, their ancestry and culture may or may not operate as a buffer against the racially pathologizing narratives that emerge in the media about African Americans.[24] However, for therapists working with Black immigrants, it is vital to capture and honor the complexity of racial identity without perpetuating an oppressive social narrative of "us versus them" in relations between Black immigrants and African Americans. Clients will benefit when counselors are sensitive to ways in which repressive institutions and processes have "been able to pit one minority group against the other."[25]

Here, therapists have a dual responsibility. On the one hand, they must examine their own positions in society, reflect on their racial identities, and consider the ways in which they interact with clients of different races. At the same time, they must continually take into account the experiences that define and shape the racial identity of their Black immigrant clients.[26]

Culturally responsive counselors recognize that when others assume an immigrant to be African American, the immigrant's Caribbean or African identity may seem diminished and become harder to represent. As the client negotiates the path through racism, they may struggle with feelings of worry, loneliness, and uncertainty. Black immigrants who can connect with African Americans may find a space to talk about their experience of discrimination in the United States, while connecting with other Black immigrants may help them discuss their native culture and the challenges of living in a new nation.

The well-being of Black immigrants in the United States is critically dependent on their ability to retain contacts with family and friends back home. As part of developing and maintaining social support, clinicians can help clients set objectives to improve communication with friends and family in their country of origin. However, immigrants may find that family members who are unfamiliar with life in the United States cannot provide the support they need, and clinicians may need to help clients get through these interactions and deal with the resulting feelings of isolation. Finding alternative support networks in the community might be helpful for clients who are socially isolated or have fallen out of touch with their families. A counselor's support and cultural responsiveness to these issues can validate an immigrant client's experience in the United States and open doors for affirming their dual status, buffering racism's effects, and building relationships with others based on shared experiences.[27]

Issues in African Assimilation to Race in America

For African immigrants, the dual status of being foreign-born and Black—combined with the poor media depictions of Black Africa—heightens one's susceptibility to racism and prejudice. The effects of prejudice are significant and detrimental. Researchers examining the effects of social exclusion on the mental health and social well-being of African immigrants in the United States found that social exclusion was associated with increased symptoms of depression and anxiety, decreased trust in society, increased isolation, and increased safety concerns. The research underscores the necessity of provider interventions that address discriminatory and structurally exclusionary processes in order to help improve the emotional and social well-being of African immigrants.[28]

The risk for social exclusion increases for African immigrants who identify as Muslim or Middle Eastern/North African; are second-generation immigrants; or have poor health. The research also shows that a higher level of income serves as a protective factor against social and economic exclusion, but higher levels of education were associated with greater experiences of sociocultural exclusion.[29]

Although factors such as education are typically protective for immigrants, in this case one's education can actually increase the risk for social exclusion and lead to higher levels of acculturative stress. Counselors may be able to help African immigrant clients think about appropriate ways to challenge exclusionary practices, create bridges between their heritage culture and their host culture, and increase their social support system.[30]

Issues in Afro-Caribbean Assimilation to Race in America

For Caribbean immigrants it is common to hold onto some of the significant customs and beliefs from one's indigenous culture while also assimilating into American society.[31] Often, Caribbean ethnicity is a significant social identity that, when joined with race, gender, sexual orientation, religion, and other identities, defines the social and cultural being of an individual.

Like African immigrants, Black Caribbean immigrants are frequently assumed to be African Americans, a presumption that ignores the fact that African-descended people in the Caribbean have cultures and histories that are distinctly different from that of African Americans.[32] While Afro-Caribbeans and African Americans both have a history of chattel slavery, slaves who lived in the Caribbean kept many aspects of their African culture. African slaves in the Caribbean came from "a polyglot of communities, linguistic groups, towns, and ethnic groups in Africa."[33] As people struggled to make sense of their newly changed lives and shared destiny, the blending of these distinct African civilizations gave rise to a unique Creole culture.[34] The music, dancing, cuisine, architecture, entrepreneurial spirit, vibrant culture, and various remnants of other African traditions may all be found throughout the Caribbean islands.

As a member of the majority population in their native island, Black Caribbeans did not face the same levels of racism and systematic marginalization as African Americans in the United States.[35] Coming to the United States, Black Caribbean immigrants are now confronted with the reality that they may be judged and devalued because of their skin color. This new and sudden experience of prejudicial treatment based on both skin color and immigrant status can be jarring.[36] All of this may be overlooked by counselors who do not understand the culturally specific experiences of Black Caribbean immigrants or the identity shifting and cultural consolidation process that may ensue. In the absence of culturally responsive care, Black Caribbean immigrants may terminate counseling early or avoid counseling completely.

Finding a Place

Whether African or Afro-Caribbean, Black immigrants from nations where their ethnic identity is not minoritized, stigmatized, or racialized find it difficult to adapt to the caste-like structure of racial identification in the United States. Their countries of origin do not employ racial classification as a social marker. By contrast, in the United States race is a person's master status and racial identity influences everything from interpersonal engagement to institutional involvement and resource distribution. As a result, many Black immigrant families find themselves reevaluating their own views on race[37] because being labeled as African American brings about an emotional and social burden from America's history of Black/White tension and social stratification. In this system, finding one's position can be intimidating and discouraging. Counselors may find clients questioning or rethinking their decision to come to the United States after encountering racism, microaggressions, or discrimination.

To find a level of comfort, Black immigrants are frequently faced with two options. They can choose to align with their ethnic group, which potentially places them in a disadvantageous and socially inferior position in American society, or they can intentionally distance themselves from US–born Blacks to attain a greater level of protection and differentiation from negative African American stereotypes and bias.[38]

African and Afro-Caribbean communities have sprung up all across the United States as a response to racial discrimination and a sense of isolation. Referred to as "enclaves," these groups form in order to preserve ethnic identities and cultural norms.[39] Members of large Afro-Caribbean enclaves may originate from a variety of islands, yet they often maintain a unified cultural identity.[40] Similar communities such as Nigerian American, Liberian American, and Ghanaian American sectors in large urban areas provide much-needed cultural connections for African immigrant families to live, work, worship, and socialize together.

Black immigrants' experiences as members of a racialized group in the United States are ameliorated, at least temporarily, by being a part of an enclave with others who share the same heritage.[41] The enclaves allow community members to more fully express their ethnic and cultural identities. However, scholars have pointed out that the "invisibility" of people within these enclaves frequently leads to increased marginalization.[42]

IMMIGRATION OVER-ENFORCEMENT

Law enforcement inequities throughout the country extend into the immigration detention system.[43] Immigration and Customs Enforcement (ICE) was created as a direct response to the September 11, 2001, terrorist attacks and was tasked with investigating, capturing, and detaining or deporting anyone suspected of breaking US immigration and customs laws.[44] Racial differences in ICE's treatment of immigrants are evident from the statistics: Black immigrants are at a measurable disadvantage.

Black immigrants make up roughly 50 percent of ICE arrests, and they are detained and deported at disproportionately greater rates than other groups.[45] Data from the Refugee and Immigrant Center for Education and Legal Services (RAICES) shows that compared to other immigrant groups, Black immigrants are three times more likely to be imprisoned for alleged criminal conduct. RAICES also found that while Black immigrants make up just 7 percent of the non-citizen population in the United States, they make up 20 percent of the immigrant population awaiting deportation. In contrast to their non–Black immigrant peers, Black African Nationals and Afro-Caribbean immigrants are six times more likely to be held in solitary confinement while detained by ICE.[46]

Forty-four percent of the families housed in ICE detention facilities during the COVID-19 pandemic in 2020 were immigrants from Haiti. The Haitian detainees have faced massive disparities in the bond amounts required for release, making it more difficult for them to gain their freedom. Between 2018 and 2020, the overall average immigration bond was $10,500, but the average bond for Haitian immigrants was $16,170.[47]

Between 2001 and 2017, the Open Policing Project at Stanford University reviewed ninety-three million traffic stops from twenty-one state patrol agencies and twenty-nine police departments and found that Black drivers are 20 percent more likely to be stopped than White drivers.[48] Laws such as the 287(g) Program, which allows local law enforcement to transfer detained immigrants to ICE custody, cause more Black immigrants to wind up in ICE's custody, with many facing deportation for minor infractions.[49]

These types of disparities have long-term stress effects on the mental and emotional health of Black immigrants. At one point, they were optimistic that coming to the United States would bring them freedom, liberty, and a better quality of life, but their lived realities often look much different. While public attention is widely given to Latinx immigration issues, it is easy to overlook the reality that Black immigrants can also live in fear for themselves and their loved ones due to potential ICE interventions. In response to those stressors, Black immigrants may be even less likely to seek professional mental health treatment than African Americans.

THE INTERSECTION OF MENTAL HEALTH AND PSYCHOSOCIAL FACTORS

Researchers who examined differences between African Americans, African immigrants, and Afro-Caribbean immigrants in the areas of mental health service utilization, medical mistrust, depression severity, mental health knowledge, and stigmatizing behavior toward people with mental illness found nuances for each sociocultural variation. Below are some highlights of that study's findings on medical mistrust, depression severity, and stigmatization.[50]

Medical Mistrust

Many Blacks in America have a justifiable mistrust of the medical community, but mistrust by African Americans is slightly higher than that felt by Black immigrants. Within the Black immigrant community, those with US citizenship reported lower levels of medical mistrust, while individuals who were not citizens indicated greater levels of mistrust. It is possible that differences in the historical narratives of African Americans and Black immigrants contribute to variations in their levels of trust. Specifically, differences in trust—based on race and citizenship status—may be a reflection of how racism in the United States has been experienced. Migration and acculturation stress, for instance, may increase skepticism of official health care institutions among non–US citizens.

Depression Severity

Differences in the level of depression severity reported by African Americans and Black immigrants are worth noting. African Americans are more likely to report moderate to severe depressive symptoms, while Black immigrants are more likely to report lower levels of depression. Understanding these differences requires looking at lived experiences, cultural explanations, epigenetic transmission, symptom interpretation, and other factors. Providers of mental health and primary care alike need to consider these distinctions and examine the client's self-reported severity as they conduct assessments and interventions with clients.

Stigmatizing Behavior

Stigmatizing behavior is the avoidance of or discomfort around others who suffer from mental illness. African Americans who had more severe depession reported experiencing more stigmatizing behavior than those with less severe symptoms. Black immigrants reported even higher levels of stigma than African Americans. The experience of stigmatizing behavior is a contributor to psychological distress and a barrier to seeking mental health services. Therefore, it is critical to address stigma, and the adverse effects of delaying treatment, especially for those suffering more serious illness.

SEE PEOPLE THE WAY THEY WANT TO BE SEEN

Providers in mental health and primary care centers have an obligation to learn more about the unique perspectives and mental health care needs of Black adults, but this demographic should not be considered a monolithic group. Providers must factor in each group's cultural distinctions to avoid making generalizations and assuming similarities that lack accuracy. Culturally responsive care requires a nuanced lens. Let us commit to using that lens to see all people of the African diaspora as they desire to be seen.

NOTES

1. bell hooks, *Salvation: Black People and Love*, reprint (New York, NY: Harper Collins / William Morrow Paperbacks, 2001).

2. *Merriam-Webster*, s.v. "diaspora (*n.*)," accessed March 20, 2023, https://www.merriam -webster.com/dictionary/diaspora.

3. Lizzie Wade, "Genetic Study Reveals Surprising Ancestry of Many Americans," Science.org, December 18, 2014, https://www.science.org/content/article/genetic-study -reveals-surprising-ancestry-many-americans.

4. Kay Deaux et al. "Becoming American: Stereotype Threat Effects in Afro-Caribbean Immigrant Groups," *Social Psychology Quarterly* 70, no. 4 (2007): 384–404, https://doi.org /10.1177/019027250707000408; Schekeva P. Hall and Robert T. Carter, "The Relationship Between Racial Identity, Ethnic Identity, and Perceptions of Racial Discrimination in an Afro-Caribbean Descent Sample," *Journal of Black Psychology* 32, no. 2 (May 2006): 155–175, https://doi.org/10.1177/0095798406287071; Violet M. Showers Johnson, "'What, Then, Is the African American?' African and Afro-Caribbean Identities in Black America," *Journal of American Ethnic History* 28, no. 1 (October 1, 2008): 77–103, https: //doi.org/10.2307/27501883; Reuel R. Rogers, "Race-Based Coalitions among Minority Groups: Afro-Caribbean Immigrants and African-Americans in New York City," *Urban Affairs Review* 39, no. 3 (2004): 283–317, https://doi.org/10.1177/1078087403258960.

5. Mary C. Waters, *Black Identities: West Indian Immigrant Dreams and American Realities* (Harvard University Press, 2009); McKalah Hudlin, "All Skinfolk Ain't Kinfolk: Examining Diasporic Differences Along Dimensions of Black Identity," (thesis, Princeton University, 2020).

6. Tony Brown et al., "Race, Nativity, Ethnicity, and Cultural Influences in the Sociology of Mental Health," in *Handbook of the Sociology of Mental Health*, eds. Carol S. Aneshensel, Jo C. Phelan, and Alex Bierman (New York: Springer, 2013), 25–76.

7. Henry Louis Gates and Donald Yacovone, *The African Americans: Many Rivers to Cross* (Carlsbad, CA: SmileyBooks, 2016).

8. Johannes Bohacek et al., "Transgenerational Epigenetic Effects on Brain Functions," *Biological Psychiatry* 73, no. 4 (2013): 313–320, https://doi.org/10.1016/j.biopsych.2012.08.019.

9. Tori Rodriguez, "Descendants of Holocaust Survivors Have Altered Stress Hormones," *Scientific American Mind* 26, no. 2 (March 1, 2015): 10–10, 10.1038/scientificamericanmind0315-10a.

10. Gates and Yacovone, *The African Americans*, 2016.

11. Monica Anderson, "African Immigrant Population in U.S. Steadily Climbs," Pew Research Center, Washington D.C. (February 14, 2017), https://www.pewresearch.org/fact-tank/2017/02/14/african-immigrant-population-in-u-s-steadily-climbs.

12. Christine Tamir and Monica Anderson, "One-in-Ten Black People Living in the U.S. Are Immigrants," Pew Research Center, Washington D.C. (January 20, 2022), https://www.pewresearch.org/race-ethnicity/2022/01/20/one-in-ten-black-people-living-in-the-u-s-are-immigrants.

13. Anderson, "African Immigrant Population," n.p.

14. Christine Tamir, "Key Findings About Black immigrants in the U.S.," Pew Research Center, January 27, 2022, https://www.pewresearch.org/fact-tank/2022/01/27/key-findings-about-black-immigrants-in-the-u-s.

15. Tamir, "Key Findings," n.p.

16. Tamir, "Key Findings," n.p.

17. Tamir and Anderson, "One-in-Ten," n.p.

18. Jane Lorenzi and Jeanne Batalova, "Sub-Saharan African Immigrants in the United States," Migrationpolicy.org, May 11, 2022, https://www.migrationpolicy.org/article/sub-saharan-african-immigrants-united-states.

19. Ogbonnaya I. Omenka, Dennis P. Watson, and Hugh C. Hendrie, "Understanding the Healthcare Experiences and Needs of African Immigrants in the United States: A Scoping Review," *BMC Public Health* 20, no. 27 (January 8, 2020), https://doi.org/10.1186/s12889-019-8127-9.

20. Bertranna Alero Muruthi et al., "'First Thing When I Walk through the Door, I Am a Black Woman': Pilot Study Examining Afro-Caribbean Women's Racial and Ethnic Identity," *Journal of Systemic Therapies* 40, no. 1 (2021): 75–91, https://doi.org/10.1521/jsyt.2021.40.1.75.

21. Muruthi et al, "First Thing."

22. Timothy J. Owens and Richard T. Serpe, "The Role of Self-Esteem in Family Identity Salience and Commitment among Blacks, Latinos, and Whites," in *Advances in Identity Theory and Research*, ed. P. J. Burke et al. (Kluwer Academic/Plenum Publishers, 2003), 85–102.

23. Muruthi et al, "First Thing."

24. Gene Combs and Jill Freedman, "Narrative Therapy's Relational Understanding of Identity," *Family Process* 55, no. 2 (May 2016): 211–24, https://doi.org/10.1111/famp.12216.

25. Cynthia Cannon Poindexter and Deborah P. Valentine, "An Introduction to Human Services: Values, Methods, and Populations Served," in *An Introduction to Human Services: Values, Methods, and Populations Served* (Boston, MA: Cengage Publishers, 2013), 30.

26. Muruthi et al, "First Thing."

27. Muruthi et al, "First Thing."

28. Sherinah Saasa and J. Lloyd Allen, "Social Exclusion among African Immigrants in the United States," *Social Work Research* 45, no. 1 (March 2021): 51–62, https://doi.org/10.1093/swr/svaa022.

29. Saasa and Allen, "Social Exclusion."

30. Saasa and Allen, "Social Exclusion."

31. David A. Baptiste, Jr., Kenneth V. Hardy, and Laurie Lewis, *Contemporary Family Therapy* 19, no. 3 (1997): 337–59, https://doi.org/10.1023/A:1026112126048; Eleanor J. Murphy and Ramaswami Mahalingam, "Transnational Ties and Mental Health of Caribbean Immigrants," *Journal of Immigrant Health* 6 (October 2004): 167–78, https://doi.org/10.1023/B:JOIH.0000045254.71331.5e.

32. Sharon-ann Gopaul-McNicol, "Caribbean Families: Social and Emotional Problems," *Journal of Social Distress and the Homeless* 7 (January 1998): 55–73, https://doi.org/10.1023/A:1022918715603; Reuel R. Rogers, *Afro-Caribbean Immigrants and the Politics of Incorporation: Ethnicity, Exception, or Exit* (Cambridge, MA: Cambridge University Press, 2006); M. C. Waters, *Black Identities*.

33. M. C. Waters, *Black Identities*, 21.

34. M. C. Waters, *Black Identities*, 21.

35. Andrew D. Case and Carla D. Hunter, "Cultural Racism–Related Stress in Black Caribbean Immigrants," *Journal of Black Psychology* 40, no. 5 (2013): 410–23, https://doi.org/10.1177/009579841349392; Hall and Carter, "The Relationship between Racial Identity."

36. Murphy and Mahalingam, "Transnational Ties."

37. Akosua Adomako Ampofo, Josephine Beoku-Betts, and Mary Johnson Osirim, "Researching African Women and Gender Studies: New Social Science Perspectives," *African and Asian Studies* 7, no. 4 (2008): 327–41, https://doi.org/10.1163/156921008X359560.

38. Johnson, "'What, Then, Is the African American?.'"

39. M. Halter, "Encyclopedia of Diasporas: Immigrant and Refugee Cultures around the World," ed. Carol R. Ember, Melvin Ember, and Ian A. Skoggard, *Encyclopedia of Diasporas: Immigrant and Refugee Cultures around the World* (New York: Kluwer Academic/Plenum, 2005), 615–23.

40. Tracey Reynolds, "Caribbean Second-Generation Return Migration: Transnational Family Relationships with 'Left-behind' Kin in Britain," *Mobilities* 6, no. 4 (2011): 535–51, https://doi.org/10.1080/17450101.2011.603946.

41. Janel E. Benson, "Exploring the Racial Identities of Black Immigrants in the United States," *Sociological Forum* 21, no. 2 (August 15, 2006): 219–47, https://doi

.org/10.1007/s11206-006-9013-7; M. L. Stephenson, "Tourism, Racism and the UK Afro-Caribbean Diaspora," in *Tourism, Diasporas and Space*, ed. Tim Coles and Dallen J. Timothy (London: Routledge, 2004), 62–77; Milton Vickerman, "Jamaicans: Balancing Race and Ethnicity," ed. N Foner, *New Immigrants in New York*, 2001, 201–28, https://doi .org/10.7312/fone92136-008; M. C. Waters, *Black Identities*.

42. Laurine Thomas, Thomas Clarke, and Alice Kroliczak, "Implementation of Peer Support Demonstration Project for HIV+ Caribbean Immigrants: A Descriptive Paper," *Journal of Immigrant & Refugee Studies* 6, no. 4 (December 18, 2008): 526–44, https://doi .org/10.1080/15362940802480407.

43. The Refugee and Immigrant Center for Education and Legal Services, "Black Immigrant Lives Are under Attack," *RAICES*, 2020, https://www.raicestexas.org/2020 /07/22/black-immigrant-lives-are-under-attack.

44. Ron Nixon and Linda Qiu, "What Is Ice and Why Do Critics Want to Abolish It?" *New York Times*, July 3, 2018, https://www.nytimes.com/2018/07/03/us/politics/fact -check-ice-immigration-abolish.html.

45. Juan Carlos Gomez and Vanessa Merez, "Immigrant Families during the Pandemic: On the Frontlines but Left Behind," CLASP (The Center for Law and Social Policy), April 1, 2022, https://www.clasp.org/publications/report/brief/immigrant-families -pandemic-frontlines.

46. The Refugee and Immigrant Center for Education and Legal Services, "Black Immigrant Lives."

47. The Refugee and Immigrant Center for Education and Legal Services, "Black Immigrant Lives."

48. The Refugee and Immigrant Center for Education and Legal Services, "Black Immigrant Lives."

49. The Refugee and Immigrant Center for Education and Legal Services, "Black Immigrant Lives."

50. Aderonke Bamgbose Pederson, Devan Hawkins, and Lynette Lartey, "Differences in Psychosocial Factors of Mental Health in an Ethnically Diverse Black Adult Population," *Journal of Public Health Policy* 43, no. 4 (2022): 670–84, https://doi.org/10.1057/ s41271-022-00379-1. This is the source for all the information under the subhead: The Intersection of Mental Health and Psychosocial Factors.

CHAPTER 3

So Many Shades of Black

Colorism and Hypodescent

One day our descendants will think it incredible that we paid so much attention to things like the amount of melanin in our skin or the shape of our eyes or our gender instead of the unique identities of each of us as complex human beings.

—FRANKLIN THOMAS

Light-skinned, fair-skinned, brown-skinned, dark-skinned, redbone, brown bone, high yellow, chocolate, ebony, waffle-colored, brown sugar, mixed, mulatto, café au lait. The variety of skin tones among African American people are described by a wide range of vernacular phrases.[1] Some of these expressions are outdated and even offensive; others are still commonly used in various contexts among African Americans. The intent here is not to delve into the interpretation or appropriateness of these color labels, but to show the degree of attention paid to skin color variances in African American culture.

COLORISM: INTRA-RACIAL AND INTERRACIAL STRATIFICATION
Skin tone has been found to be a significant predictor of life outcomes for Black people—a large body of research bears this out.[2] This has been the case since the beginning of colonialism. It is known as colorism.

When people of African ancestry experience discrimination because they are Black, that is a form of racism. However, when the degree of discrimination varies based on the lightness or darkness of a person's skin tone, this is *colorism*—the socialization of skin tone—which is a subset of race-based bias.[3] The term, which was coined in the early 1980s and is credited to Pulitzer Prize–winning author Alice Walker, refers to the preferential treatment given to people with lighter skin and other Eurocentric standards of beauty. Walker addressed this internalized and inherently divisive preference among Black people as an outcome of socialization that values the physical traits of European descent more than those of African descent.[4]

Racism and colorism are two separate but related phenomena. The ideology and aesthetics of White superiority rely on the persistent stereotype that people with lighter complexions are more refined and cultured than those with darker skin, and that those with darker color are more barbaric, illogical, ugly, and inferior. These views are the bedrock of colorism.[5]

Greater amounts of melanin production mean darker skin pigmentation and devalued appearance, making darker complexions the targets of intergroup and intragroup stigmatization.[6] Historically, people with darker skin tones have had higher levels of stigma consciousness and the expectation of being stereotyped. The mere anticipation of being typecast can have a detrimental impact on both the life satisfaction and mental health of African Americans.[7]

The origins of African American skin color stratification can be traced back to slavery. The broad range of skin tones among African American people is evidence of the White ancestry intergenerationally woven throughout the bloodline. In the United States, the slave trade was a culture of rape wherein White slave owners and overseers used sexual violence for social control and to expand their unpaid work force. The law said that a single drop of Black blood categorized a person as Black. Therefore, multiracial infants born to enslaved mothers were legally identified as Black, so they were enslaved even though their fathers were White.

These young slaves had lighter skin tones and frequently more White ancestral traits than Black traits. It was here that the stratification of skin tone within Black racialization commenced. Along with this stratification emerged a hierarchy of color and privilege. These lighter-skinned children were still slaves, but they frequently had more specialized labor assignments, easier workloads, inside assignments rather than arduous fieldwork, and even more leniency in earning their way to freedom. Such were the privileges afforded to people with lighter complexion and naturally straighter hair, while those with darker skin, wider noses, and tightly curled hair were considered unsightly and even barbaric.

Embracing *every* drop is a challenge when you are indelibly defined by just *one* drop.

African Americans have continued to live in a highly stratified socioeconomic structure in which those with lighter complexion have advantages in terms of wealth, education, and occupational reputation. Those with lighter skin tones report greater levels of education and occupational prestige and are more likely to have spouses with higher levels of education and employment.[8]

Some organizations engaged in blatant intra-racial colorism into the early 1900s: Upper-class African American groups or businesses would conduct a skin-color test using a brown paper bag. If a person's skin tone was darker than the paper bag, they were deemed to be too dark and were refused membership or entrance. Today, African Americans recognize this archaic behavior as dishonorable, offensive, and polarizing.

By the end of the baby boom, skin tone disparities had slightly less significance for educational and occupational success, but still had an impact on marriage choice and spousal social status, as light skin tone was seen as more attractive, refined, socially acceptable, and upwardly mobile.

Lighter-skinned African American women had better educational attainment and personal earnings than darker-skinned African American women, and they were also more likely to marry males with higher educational attainments.

Research has also shown a significant correlation between European standards of beauty and the perception of competence. Whether evaluated intra-racially or interracially, a lighter complexion was linked to perceived capacity, intellect, and responsibility. Even after controlling for other factors associated with discrimination, in-group colorism is a significant risk factor for worse physical health among African Americans.[9]

The Black community has a saying, "The blacker the berry, the sweeter the juice," which is meant to be a positive affirmation of darker complexions and works to counteract the idealization of lighter skin tones by recognizing the beauty in deeper melanin. Another saying, "Black don't crack," means that dark skin does not age as quickly as lighter skin. The phrase "Black is beautiful" became well known in the early 1960s as part of a campaign to challenge the exclusivity of White beauty. These affirmations highlight the positive attributes and attractiveness of Black skin to counter the emphasis on White standards of beauty.

SKIN TONE AND FAMILY DYNAMICS

Researchers have begun to examine race, ethnicity, and colorism in family processes such as parenting.[10] The range of genetic and phenotypic expressions in a Black family produces a wide variety of complexions, even among siblings who share the same two parents. Colorism was discovered to affect how family members treated children, with lighter-skinned children receiving preferential treatment over those with darker complexions.

Qualitative research on the role of Black families in creating skin tone bias discovered that families are the most significant influence on how people perceive themselves and others in terms of skin tone.[11] Studies show varying effects. Nancy Boyd Franklin proposed that some parents with dark-skinned children may scapegoat them while elevating their lighter-skinned offspring above their siblings.[12] On the other hand, some parents may provide extra assistance to their darker-skinned children because they perceive their child's skin tone as a social liability.[13] Research points to the reality of people with darker complexions facing more racial prejudice,[14] so parents may use their parenting style to combat racism or shield their children from racial prejudice.[15]

Counselors must not overlook the fact that Black processes of racial socialization in families (teaching children what it means to be a member of their race) is affected by skin tone. Antoinette Landor and colleagues found that parenting styles based on complexion in families also tend to vary based on the child's gender. In Landor's study, children rated their parents' quality of parenting. Dark-skinned males rated their parents more highly than males with lighter skin tones, while daughters with lighter skin reported the experience of higher quality parenting than those with darker skin tones.[16]

The reasons for these differences are complex. For sons, parents know—and research supports—the reality that the color of a Black man's skin affects his life. Those with darker skin are at a disadvantage in education, income, and the job market. With this awareness, parents of boys with darker skin may strive to combat those social inequities by investing more parental time and energy in those children to help set them up for greater success.[17] With the survival of darker-skinned sons front and center, Black parents also tend to give darker-skinned sons more messages promoting mistrust of others than they give to sons with lighter skin.[18]

For daughters, however, Landor found that the psychology of parenting appears to be different, and thus the parenting effects are reversed. Lighter-skinned daughters reported that they received higher-quality parenting than those with darker skin, which is consistent with research findings that show preferential treatment of family members with lighter skin. Because of the White standards of beauty valued most by society, a lighter skin tone becomes a type of social capital for Black women. Parents may have consciously or unconsciously internalized this gendered colorism and thereby demonstrate a greater quality of parenting to their lighter-skinned daughters.[19]

The skin tone of the primary caregiver is a notable variable as well. Darker skin parents instill more messages of mistrust to their adolescent daughters than lighter skin parents do. Conversely, lighter skin parents of adolescent sons provide more mistrust messages than darker skin parents. Counselors, therefore, must not overlook this particular paradox of race.

The reality is that while Black parents are intentional about delivering racial socialization messages that can help buffer or shield children from the effects of racism, they may also unintentionally perpetuate colorism.[20]

THE CHALLENGES OF BIRACIAL AND MULTIRACIAL IDENTITIES

Mia is a graduate student pursuing a master's degree in counseling. She wrote a personal race narrative for her diversity counseling course:

I always stare at the race boxes longer than I should when filling out forms. What do I pick? What are the rules for mixed kids? My mother is Colombian and Italian. My father describes himself as "Afro-Rican" but to put it plainly, he is Puerto Rican and African American.

So, I am 1/4 White, 1/4 African American, 1/4 Columbian, and 1/4 Puerto Rican, and I appear physically as Hispanic. When I stare at the race boxes on a form and must pick only one, I usually choose White. I don't choose Black because I don't think I look Black, so I feel like an imposter choosing that one. If I can check two boxes, I check White and Black. When I distill it all down, I am a person of mixed race and ethnically I am Hispanic.

For a very long time, I thought my race and my Hispanic ethnicity were something to hide and be ashamed of. In elementary and middle school, I used to lie and say I was White and only a fourth Hispanic. I had this whole story that my grandfather was the only one who wasn't White in my family and that's how I got the last name Sanchez. I was embarrassed and mad that I wasn't White. I feel so sad for the younger Mia. She lied about her race and ethnicity to try to fit into the predominantly White spaces around her. She used to get angry when people asked, "What are you?" and she felt the need to defend and protect herself. I'm not a "what" at all!

Growing up, my family did not talk about race or ethnicity. Even though we were a blended, multiracial family, we grew up never addressing what that meant. I knew my mom was half Colombian because she would cook us Colombian food, but we didn't talk about what that meant either. I don't have a single memory of my family talking about race or ethnicity other than my mom calling me her "brown child" because I was the tannest out of my sisters. I knew my dad was mixed but it seemed like the most important thing about him was that he was from New York. Both my parents struggled with being mixed growing up, so I think their plan for us was to just not address it and hope we grew up without thinking about our race and ethnicity. I believe this contributed to my rejection of the Hispanic and Black parts of me. I saw it as something to avoid and brush under the rug. All I knew was that my family looked very different from other families.

As an undergraduate student in college, I finally started to become more comfortable with who I was and what I looked like. I stopped lying and although I still struggle with feeling like an imposter because I don't know much about my cultures, I know that doesn't invalidate my ethnicity or race. Every day, I am working to embrace every drop of me!

Just One Drop

Embracing *every* drop is a challenge when you are indelibly defined by just *one* drop. The "one-drop rule," or "hypodescent," is the basis of the conventional American racial paradigm.[21] The one-drop rule is based on a Virginia statute from 1662 that established legal guidelines for the treatment of people of mixed race. If a person had even one remote Black ancestor, that individual would be considered Black. Even in recent decades, hypodescent has been upheld: a Louisiana court declared in 1985 that a woman whose great-great-great-great grandmother was Black must be classified as Black. With an ancestry that was 97 percent White, the state categorized the woman as Black and prohibited her from identifying as White on legal documents.[22]

Until the year 2000, people could only identify their race using one of the limited boxes on the US Census form. The choices available in 2000 changed how a large number of Americans self-identified, as more than seven million people checked more than one option when asked to identify their racial heritage. In 2010, about nine million people chose more than one option. As a result of further modifications to the census questions for 2020, there were 338 million people who identified as multiracial in the US Census, a 276 percent rise from the previous decade.

The US Census Bureau cautions that the comparisons of data between 2010 and 2020 likely reflect two different types of change. First, advances in questions and coding offer the opportunity for respondents to describe themselves with improved accuracy. Second, there are real changes in population reflected in the 2020 reporting. Within the realm of racially defined groupings, growth was notable in monoracial as well as multiracial communities. The nation saw an increase of 29 percent in the number of people who self-identified as belonging to "Some Other Race" alone or "Some Other Race in Combination," for a total of 49.9 million people choosing these options.

Between 2010 and 2020, the population of people who identify as Black/African American alone increased by 5.6 percent.[23] The total number of people who identify as Black/African American in combination with another race increased by 88.7 percent.[24] In 2020, almost 47 million people identified as being either Black/African American or Black/African American in conjunction with another race group.[25] For others, the one-drop rule influences racial socialization in such a way that many biracial people still feel obligated to primarily identify with their most minoritized race, despite having parents or grandparents from two or more racial or ethnic backgrounds.

Research beyond the census reports shows that the legacy of African Americans involves broad genetic admixture with DNA inherited from multiple populations. Genome-wide ancestry estimates for African Americans show average proportions of 73.2 percent African, 24 percent European, and 0.8 percent Native American ancestry.[26] The same study estimates that initial admixture between Europeans and Native Americans occurred twelve generations ago, followed by subsequent African admixture six generations ago. Additional studies show a gender trend in African American ancestry, with greater European male and African female representations.[27] These findings add to the narrative of slavery as a rape culture where enslaved women were violated by slaveholders who then regarded their own offspring as inferior under the one-drop rule.

In our diversity-conscious environment, clients are talking to counselors about their racial background and ethnic identity more than ever before. Consider the case of R. J., a millennial mixed-race (Black and White) male. R. J. came to counseling because of the relationship strain between him and the White family who adopted him in his infancy: "They [family members] want me to just see the world through their White lens, but even though I grew up in a White environment, I connect more with Black culture." R. J. says his adoptive parents have tried to deny him opportunities to experience and own his African American heritage: "I was light skinned so they thought they could raise me as White. They live in a White bubble and expect me to do the same thing." He says his parents always told him to stay away from certain neighborhoods because of "bad influences," which really meant "Black people." R. J. explained to his counselor that his family doesn't comprehend the experience of racism, or their own biases, so they reject his viewpoint. R.J. told his counselor, "They believe I should cut off my locs," as he pointed to his natural hair twists. "Just pass for White without having to deal with all the issues of being a Black man. They act like I should be f——ing grateful, but I do *not* want to pass for White!"

PASSING

Because of the one-drop rule, Black phenotypic expression spans a broad spectrum of skin tones, hair textures, body shapes, and facial features. For decades, biracial Americans constituted a larger proportion of the US population than was recognized, beause with the right combination of phenotypic features, some biracial people were able to pass for White.

Because the rule of hypodescent made it illegal for a person of multiple races to identify as White, doing so was quite risky. Those who chose to pass for White acquired access to the freedoms and opportunities of Whiteness but found it necessary to disavow their Black identity and pose as monoracial individuals. However, if the White community discovered a person passing as White, that person faced serious consequences or even death.

African American communities have historically had mixed reactions to passing. In the past, passing frequently involved transferring to a new location to begin their new life as a White person. This often meant moving to a larger city where no one would know about their "deception." These relocations were often initiated by parents when their light-skinned children were old enough to live independently. Family members accepted that their only future contact would be if their loved one secretly returned to the family home, because traveling to see them in their new environment would risk revealing the secret of their true racial identity. They believed this was the best option for their son or daughter's survival and for protection against the ills of a racist society.

Other African American people saw passing as a selfish betrayal of one's own race, which created familial discord and even estrangement. Those who passed frequently lost family and friends. Dating and marrying a White person typically meant keeping their identity a secret even from their spouse. So, they missed going home for family gatherings for holidays, graduations, family reunions, weddings, and their parents' funerals. Passing can be compared to going underground in a witness protection program, but having no protection. They lost the ability to honestly answer normal questions such as "Where are you from?" or "Who are your people?" A person who chose to pass could never "come out" as Black. Keshia Harris suggests that crossing the "color line" in this way was another form of "privilege given to biracial individuals who are able to identify with their European American heritge and hide their minority status" because their appearance was racially ambiguous.[28]

In the case of R. J., he refused to follow the advice of his adoptive parents who wanted him to pass. Passing is now seen as a rather archaic notion. However, ancestral genetic testing is revealing lineage and introducing people to relatives of other races. The discovery of one's multiracial heritage can be met with conflicting emotions for an individual and mixed responses within a family. Counselors must not overlook the fact that as clients are able to learn more about their ancestry than ever before, the results may bring mixed feelings about the identities and the racial identification of their ancestors, and about those who hid the truth.

A counselor who is sensitive to culture supports their client's need for self-acceptance. This counselor offers help to a client who is struggling to establish a feeling of connectedness in any of their racial or ethnic origins or who feels as though they have no cultural home to call their own. The counselor might work with the client to assist them in processing race-based family conflicts and responding appropriately to those conflicts. Counselors who are culturally attentive steer clear of brushing off or downplaying the client's experiences of loneliness and isolation. Yet, in all of that, the counselor must not over-assess a client or presume that the client's work in therapy needs to be related to their racial identities. A client may be seeking counseling for problems related to any aspect of their lives, and the counselor who overlooks the other areas of a client's life may risk doing just as much harm as they would by overlooking salient racial issues. In all client considerations, counselor sensitivity is paramount.

NOTES

1. JeffriAnne Wilder, "Revisiting 'Color Names and Color Notions': A Contemporary Examination of the Language and Attitudes of Skin Color among Young Black Women," *Journal of Black Studies* 41, no. 1 (2010): 184–206, https://doi.org/10.1177/0021934709337986.

2. Travis L. Dixon and Keith B. Maddox, "Skin Tone, Crime News, and Social Reality Judgments: Priming the Stereotype of the Dark and Dangerous Black Criminal," *Journal of Applied Social Psychology* 35, no. 8 (2005): 1555–70, https://doi.org/10.1111/j.1559-1816.2005.tb02184.x; Arthur H Goldsmith, Darrick Hamilton, and William Darity, "Shades of Discrimination: Skin Tone and Wages," *American Economic Review* 96, no. 2 (May 2006): 242–45, https://doi.org/10.1257/000282806777212152; Lance Hannon, Robert DeFina, and Sarah Bruch, "The Relationship between Skin Tone and School Suspension for African Americans," *Race and Social Problems* 5, no. 4 (September 5, 2013): 281–95, https://doi.org/10.1007/s12552-013-9104-z; Joni Hersch, "Skin-Tone Effects among African Americans: Perceptions and Reality," *American Economic Review* 96, no. 2 (May 2006): 251–55, https://doi.org/10.1257/000282806777212071; Asia T McCleary-Gaddy and Drexler James, "Skin Tone, Life Satisfaction, and Psychological Distress among African Americans: The Mediating Effect of Stigma Consciousness," *Journal of Health Psychology* 27, no. 2 (2020): 422–31, https://doi.org/10.1177/1359105320954251

3. Keshia L. Harris, "Biracial American Colorism: Passing for White," *American Behavioral Scientist* 62, no. 14 (2018): 2072–86, https://doi.org/10.1177/0002764218810747.

4. Harris, "Biracial American Colorism."

5. Margaret Hunter, "The Persistent Problem of Colorism: Skin Tone, Status, and Inequality," *Sociology Compass* 1, no. 1 (September 2007): 237–54, https://doi.org/10.1111/j.1751-9020.2007.00006.x.

6. Irene V. Blair, Charles M. Judd, and Kristine M. Chapleau, "The Influence of Afrocentric Facial Features in Criminal Sentencing," *Psychological Science* 15, no. 10 (2004): 674–79, https://doi.org/10.1111/j.0956-7976.2004.00739.x; Goldsmith, Hamilton, and William Darity, "Shades of Discrimination"; Keith B. Maddox and Stephanie A. Gray, "Cognitive Representations of Black Americans: Reexploring the Role of Skin Tone," *Personality and Social Psychology Bulletin* 28, no. 2 (2002): 250–59, https://doi.org/10.1177/0146167202282010; McCleary-Gaddy and James, "Skin Tone"; Ellis P. Monk, Jr., "The Cost of Color: Skin Color, Discrimination, and Health among African-Americans," *American Journal of Sociology* 121, no. 2 (2015): 396–444, https://doi.org/10.1086/682162.

7. Elizabeth C. Pinel, "Stigma Consciousness: The Psychological Legacy of Social Stereotypes." *Journal of Personality and Social Psychology* 76, no. 1 (1999): 114–28, https://doi.org/10.1037/0022-3514.76.1.114; Monk, Jr., "The Cost of Color."

8. Verna M. Keith and Cedric Herring, "Skin Tone and Stratification in the Black Community," *American Journal of Sociology* 97, no. 3 (1991): 760–78, https://doi.org/10.1086/229819.

9. Monk, Jr., "The Cost of Color."

10. Antoinette M. Landor et al., "Exploring the Impact of Skin Tone on Family Dynamics and Race-Related Outcomes.," *Journal of Family Psychology* 27, no. 5 (2013): 817–26, https://doi.org/10.1037/a0033883.

11. JeffriAnne Wilder and Colleen Cain, "Teaching and Learning Color Consciousness in Black Families: Exploring Family Processes and Women's Experiences with Colorism," *Journal of Family Issues* 32, no. 5 (2010): 577–604, https://doi.org/10.1177/0192513x10390858.

12. Nancy Boyd-Franklin, *Black Families in Therapy: Understanding the African American Experience* (New York, NY: Guilford Press, 2003).

13. Beverly A. Greene, "Sturdy Bridges: The Role of African-American Mothers in the Socialization of African-American Children," *Women & Therapy* 10, no. 1–2 (1990): 205–25, https://doi.org/10.1300/j015v10n01_18; Landor, et al., "Exploring the Impact."

14. Elizabeth Klonniff and Hope Landrine, "Is Skin Color a Marker for Racial Discrimination? Explaining the Skin Color-Hypertension Relationship," *Journal of Behavioral Medicine* 23, no. 4 (August 1, 2000): 329–38, https://doi.org/10.1023/A:1005580300128.

15. Landor, et al., "Exploring the Impact."

16. Landor, et al., "Exploring the Impact."

17. Mark E. Hill, "Color Differences in the Socioeconomic Status of African American Men: Results of a Longitudinal Study," *Social Forces* 78, no. 4 (June 2000): 1437–60, https://doi.org/10.2307/3006180; Landor, et al., "Exploring the Impact."

18. Landor, et al., "Exploring the Impact."

19. Wilder, "Revisiting 'Color Names and Color Notions.'"; Landor, et al., "Exploring the Impact."

20. Landor, et al., "Exploring the Impact."

21. James Floyd Davis, *Who Is Black?: One Nation's Definition* (University Park, PA: Pennsylvania State Univ. Press, 1993).

22. "Defining Race," in *The Individual and Society*, accessed April 5, 2023, https://www.facinghistory.org/resource-library/defining-race.

23. Nicholas Jones et al., "2020 Census Illuminates Racial and Ethnic Composition of the Country," *Census.gov*, August 12, 2021, https://www.census.gov/library/stories/2021/08/improved-race-ethnicity-measures-reveal-united-states-population-much-more-multiracial.html.

24. Jones et al., "2020 Census Illuminates."

25. Jones et al., "2020 Census Illuminates."

26. Katarzyna Bryc et al., "The Genetic Ancestry of African Americans, Latinos, and European Americans across the United States," *The American Journal of Human Genetics* 96, no. 1 (2015): 37–53, https://doi.org/10.1016/j.ajhg.2014.11.010.

27. Joanne M. Lind et al., "Elevated Male European and Female African Contributions to the Genomes of African American Individuals," *Human Genetics* 120, no.

5 (2007): 713–22, https://doi.org/10.1007/s00439-006-0261-7; Katarzyna Bryc, et al., "The Genetic Ancestry."

28. Harris, "Biracial American Colorism."

Part II

Overlooked Historical Factors

CHAPTER 4

Down through the Years and Still through the Tears

We have come over a way that with tears has been watered,
We have come, treading our path through the blood of the slaughtered.
—JAMES WELDON JOHNSON

THESE WORDS ARE AN EXCERPT FROM THE BLACK NATIONAL ANTHEM, "Lift Every Voice and Sing." James Weldon Johnson, a poet, activist, and diplomat wrote the lyrics to the song in 1900 and the music was composed by his brother, John Rosamond Johnson.[1] The entire song is a "history lesson, a rallying cry, a pledge of unity . . . an ever-present refrain."[2] The lyrics speak profoundly to the experience of America's descendants of slavery. They speak to the history of trauma and the power of hope.

Some systems choose to overlook the impact that US history has had on the mental health and self-identity of African Americans.[3] However, from chattel slavery to today, being an African American descendant of slavery has been wrought with individual and collective traumatic experiences. This chapter provides a broad overview of trauma's effect on the African American experience and African American mental health in particular.

TRAUMA DEFINED

The Substance Abuse and Mental Health Services Administration (SAMHSA) describes individual trauma as resulting from "an event, series of events, or set of circumstances that is experienced by an individual as physically or emotionally harmful or life threatening and that has lasting adverse effects on the individual's functioning and mental, physical, social, emotional, or spiritual well-being."[4] Traumatic events often leave people feeling violated, and the symptoms a person experiences in the aftermath of those traumatic events may impair functioning, even if the person is not aware of how the event affected or influenced them.[5]

While the word "trauma" is often used to describe a life-threatening or life-altering *event,* trauma is more correctly defined as a person's *response* to a potentially tragic event that affects them or someone they care about. In this way, trauma is the body's experience. It is the *result* of being exposed to a traumatic event or set of events.

Responses to trauma are highly individual. Different people can experience the exact same event and respond differently. One person may develop symptoms of trauma, while another adjusts without experiencing any trauma response at all.

Psychologists generally accept that trauma can be caused by three levels of exposure: *acute* (a single, one-time event), *chronic* (repeated and prolonged exposure such as domestic violence or abuse), or *complex* (resulting from exposure to varied and multiple traumatic events, often of an invasive, interpersonal nature).

When trauma is experienced in the developmental years, it influences brain development and creates long-term consequences that can last for years after the traumatic event. In fact, early-life trauma can inhibit the development of neural pathways and change the brain's responses.[6] Trauma histories can cause individuals to have avoidant behaviors, numbing responses, hyperarousal, and other indicators of extreme sensitivity to the threat of danger. An individual may have problems with emotional regulation because the anticipation of harm remains dominant in the brain, making the individual less able to relax. These neurological responses are normative survival and protective reactions to abnormal circumstances.[7] They occur involuntarily for a person who has experienced trauma, but that trauma victim often will experience social stigmatization, labeling, blame, arrests, and incarceration as a result of those reflexive responses.

Trauma as a Wound

"Trauma" is the Greek word for "wound."[8] The *Merriam-Webster Dictionary* explains that the Greeks only used this term for physical injuries, but in modern interpretation, trauma also refers to emotional wounds. Physically speaking, a wound is damage to the body's tissue. Whether the wound is a bruise or a tear, the body's natural mending mechanisms are quick to get to work after any kind of injury. Psychological wounds, such as dignity loss, also bring pain. In response, the sympathetic nervous system—the brain's trauma response team—activates instantly. There is no bleeding wound or damaged skin to which the body's healing reaction may be directed, but a psychological wound such as dignity loss is a wound to the very essence of one's being.

People go to their family doctor for physical injuries. They see a counselor for emotional wounds. In counseling, racialized clients are often unaware that the wounds of their presenting issues are harder to heal because they are deeply transmitted wounds to the soul.

Historical and Intergenerational Trauma

Researchers have explored what happens when communities are exposed to catastrophic events such as war, acts of terrorism, hunger, and genocide. Studies show that trauma responses are pervasive among those populations, and the consequences of traumatic events are not restricted to firsthand experience, but are also intergenerationally transmitted.

"Historical trauma" is the term used to describe the effects of painful experiences or events that have occurred and affected a large portion of a society, or perhaps an entire community, ethnic group, or nation. Three conditions must be met to confirm historical trauma: widespread effects, collective suffering, and malicious intent.[9] By that definition, African Americans have been subjected to centuries of historical trauma.

Historical trauma response symptoms can include drug and alcohol misuse, suicidal ideations, depression, anxiety, low self-esteem, rage, violence, and trouble controlling one's emotions.[10] Societal responses are often dismissive (e.g., "Just get over it"), invalidating (e.g., "It wasn't all that bad"), devaluing (e.g., "Other cultures had slavery, too"), or detaching (e.g., "That was a long time ago"). While much of society denies that any lasting damage was done, counselors cannot afford to deny the collective burden or the unsung resilience of African Americans.

Intergenerational trauma, also known as multigenerational or trans-generational trauma, is experienced similarly but has its transmission seated in family systems: "Intergenerational trauma affects one family. While each generation of that family may experience its own form of trauma, the first experience can be traced back decades."[11] It is hypothesized that intergenerational trauma is passed down through genetic alterations in a person's DNA expression after they experience traumatic events. There is evidence supporting the notion that these genetic markers are transmitted from one generation to another. While there is no change in the DNA sequence, there appear to be changes in the DNA expression.

For example, a 1988 study of children with at least one parent or grandparent who was a Holocaust survivor found that those offspring were overrepresented in psychiatric referrals by 300 percent.[12] Additionally, a 2018 study found that the male offspring of Civil War prisoners of war (POWs) had shorter life spans than those whose fathers had not been POWs. In this study, the researchers concluded that epigenetic channels could be the mechanism through which paternal stress affects future generations. These findings provide "proof of concept" for the transmission of paternal trauma.[13] In 2005, researchers found that women who were exposed to the attack on the World Trade Center in 2001–and their infant children–had decreased levels of the hormone cortisol, which helps control the body's response to stress.[14] Similarly, a 2015 study showed that the descendants of Holocaust survivors had altered stress hormone profiles when compared to their peers.[15]

SLAVERY AND ITS INTERGENERATIONAL EFFECTS

Slavery in the United States was founded and justified on the basis of skin color and the presumption of inferiority.[16] It was an oppressive system that legally permitted the dehumanization of people of African origin.[17] Slaves were considered too inferior and uncivilized to be respected as human beings. They were treated as property to be bought, sold, branded, and killed at the will of slaveholders. By the time the Thirteenth Amendment to the US Constitution abolished slavery, it had been legally practiced for approximately three hundred years. Women were frequently raped by slavers, and men, women, and children could be beaten, lynched, burned, or killed in any manner for attempting to escape or just for declaring their own dignity.

Today, African Americans have only been out of slavery for about 160 years. The number of years that African Americans were enslaved is still nearly double the number of years that African Americans have been free. To put that timeframe into perspective, someone born the year the slaves were freed is only three generations before me. Figure 4.1 is a photo of my maternal great grandmother, born around the time slavery was being abolished. This photo speaks volumes about life for her generation in America.

The Trauma of Dignity Loss

In recent years, humiliation has been increasingly examined and recognized as a trauma-invoking way of exercising power. Philip Leask's definition of humiliation is fitting in this discussion: Humiliation is "a demonstrative exercise of power against one or more persons, which consistently involves a number of elements: stripping of status; rejection or exclusion; unpredictability or arbitrariness; and a personal sense of injustice matched by the lack of any remedy for the injustice suffered."[18]

Leask explains that humiliation comes with consistently occurring traumatic elements and consequences. Among those consequences is the inability to trust others. Power—used demonstratively, unjustly, and with cruelty—is central to humiliation. The abuse of power is demeaning and always entails rejection or exclusion.[19] Such was the experience of slavery. Yet while the historical (and sometimes contemporary) trauma of dignity loss is attached to the DNA of every descendant of slavery, a determination to survive can lead them through the societal maze of finding one's worth.

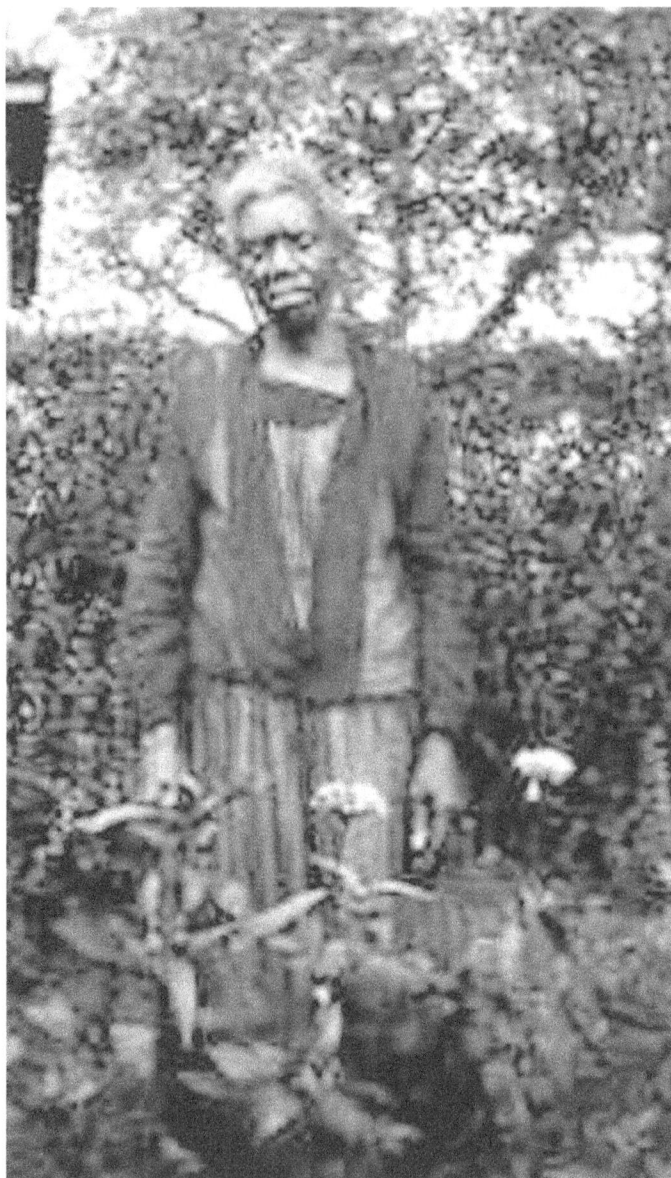

Figure 4.1 My great grandmother, Lula Osborne, born in North Carolina in the mid-1860s. The physical and emotional weathering of her body and soul are evident in her 70-year-old face and her posture in this mid 1930s photo.
SOURCE: AUTHOR'S PERSONAL COLLECTION.

The Trauma of Family Loss

The system of slavery gave the slaveholder total control over African men, women, and children who were legally recognized as property while depriving the slaves of any legal rights and autonomy. This societal structure robbed enslaved people of their right to even the most fundamental social relationship: the family. Slaves were unable to legally marry, required an owner's consent to join in non-legal unions, and could be forced to marry a partner of the owner's choosing regardless of the slave's previous relationship or marital status.

One of the most traumatizing, agonizing, and humiliating aspects of slavery was the slave auction. The institution of slavery gave no thought to familial ties. Husbands and wives had no way to avoid being sold apart from one another and were powerless to prevent their young children from being sold away from them, never to be reunited again. Slaves lived every day with the fear of being separated from children, parents, spouses, and siblings who could be sold like livestock without notice.

When a plantation owner died, it was common practice for the slaves to be sold as part of the estate, often dividing families between several buyers. The myth used to justify this blatant disregard for family was the dehumanizing idea that Africans did not have the capacity for strong kinship bonds. So, enslaved people lived daily with rage, the traumatic grief of sudden loss, and resentment of the slaveholders toward whom they could show no anger without experiencing brutal and barbaric consequences. Slaves often wanted to see their slaveholders die, but that would likely result in the sale and further separation of family members.

History texts often gloss over the misery of the forced and sudden separation of enslaved families and the tenuous hope that, with emancipation, those family members would be reunited. A few were successful in reunification. Most were not. As a result, the trauma of losing family connections runs deep in the emotional veins of African Americans.

The Trauma of Rape and Sexual Exploitation

Slavery was a culture of rape, a heinous crime that causes damage that cannot be undone. However, the rape of enslaved women was *not* considered a crime for slavers and slaveholders. Based on the broad range of skin tones seen among African Americans and the illegality of interracial marriage in most states prior to the US Supreme Court's 1967 *Loving v. Virginia* ruling, it is safe to say that most African Americans have numerous rape survivors and children of rape in their ancestral bloodlines. As Grand states, "The violence of [W]hite incursions was written, and rewritten, on their bodies, and on the skin of succeeding generations."[20]

Grand reminds us that people have offered excuses for men like Thomas Jefferson, saying that he and other slaveholders "fathered" children with their female slaves. Slave rape gets whitewashed to suggest a daring romance between slave and slaveholder. Terms like "fathering" and "mistress" suggest that a woman had the power to choose that partnership. In truth, it was not possible, as an enslaved woman, to say "no" without brutal or even fatal consequences for herself, her children, or her husband.[21]

Sexual exploitation degrades women. Adding to the trauma was the sense of emasculation, helplessness, and insult felt by enslaved men who were often forced to watch or listen, powerlessly, as their wives, daughters, and sisters were victimized. The horror of slave rape brought lasting consequences in the form of pain and blame. Author and educator bell hooks explained that "in a universe of such racial madness, this incursion of whiteness into black vaginas yielded a transgenerational legacy of shame, rage, terror and a tendency to blame the victim."[22]

The Trauma of Escape

Slaves who chose to take flight from the horrors of slavery in the southern states were considered fugitives. In general, they fled to free northern states or to Canada, but their escape came with huge risks. The journey involved the constant threat of sheriffs, limited food, little access to shelter, and avoiding slave catchers with vicious dogs, all while often traveling on foot. Slave catchers frequently placed runaway slave advertisements in newspapers and posted signs. If a runaway slave was captured, they were typically beaten and sometimes shackled; they could also be sold after they were recovered because they were deemed as rebellious. For many slaves, however, the risk was worth it. The goal was to find freedom or die trying.

The Trauma of Jim Crow Segregation

Slavery was abolished in 1865 and for a few years freed African Americans made progress with social, political, educational, and economic goals. But from the late 1800s until the Civil Rights Movement of the 1950s and 1960s, another system of control and discrimination called "Jim Crow segregation" perpetuated racist attitudes in the South with laws that controlled the lives of Black people.

State laws allowed establishments to refuse service to African American people and allowed transportation companies to limit where African American people could sit on public transportation, forcing them to the rear of the bus or separate cars on a train. There were separate water fountains, separate entrances to public establishments, separate restrooms, separate schools, separate theater seats, separate cemeteries—a full system of totalitarian racism.

For those who dared violate any of these laws, the consequences were not unlike the punishment inflicted upon rebellious slaves, up to and including lynchings and other forms of murder. Any accusation of violating Jim Crow statutes was typically a death sentence, and Whites were permitted to take the law into their own hands without allowing the accused person to have any due process under the law. In fact, in 1896, a White racist US Supreme Court ruled that Jim Crow segregation was constitutional, forcing African American men, women, and children to endure the fear and humiliation of these widespread practices.

From the end of the Civil War to the late 1940s, there are 4,084 racial terror lynchings documented in twelve Southern states. There were more than three hundred additional lynchings in states outside of the South.[23] The violent public nature of lynchings traumatized African American people, who knew they had no protection under the law in the former slave states.

Historical and intergenerational trauma is immeasurably coursing through the veins of African Americans.

Many people were lynched even without any criminal accusation. They were killed because of their anti-segregation activity, or because they took a stand for equal rights, or because of supposed minor or feigned social slights toward White people. The Equal Justice Initiative, a Montgomery-based nonprofit organization, has done extensive research on the lawless killing of Black people and summarized lynching as a way of controlling an entire race of people: "Racial terror lynching was a tool used to enforce Jim Crow laws and racial segregation—a tactic for maintaining racial control by victimizing the entire African American community, not merely punishment of an alleged perpetrator for a crime."[24]

HOW TRAUMA RESPONSES MANIFEST TODAY

Counselors must not overlook the notion that trauma creates an epigenetic signature—a chemical imprint—on an individual's genes that can be passed onto future generations. This mark does not cause a physical change in the actual genetic material, but it does modify the expression mechanism of the gene. With advances in epigenetic research, there is growing support for the idea that a person's traumatic experiences can change their biology as well as the biology and behaviors of their offspring.[25] Imagine how the extreme conditions and trauma of captivity, sexual exploitation, chattel slavery, family loss, dignity loss, escape attempts, and Jim Crow segregation affected the biology of enslaved people and their offspring.

The "antisocial" label gets cast upon traumatized African Americans who live, work, and socialize in systems that are quite often antisocial toward *them*. Behaviors such as aggression, hyperactivity, and poor impulse control are often automatic responses to threats. The medical treatment system categorizes these threat responses as pathological or externalizing behaviors. The legal system categorizes the behaviors as deviant and criminal. Social systems treat the behaviors as antisocial. The educational system categorizes the behaviors as disruptive, defiant, or learning disabled. Counseling often focuses on anger management or replacing aggressive behavior with verbal communication skills.

Rarely do any of these systems recognize the effects of current, day-to-day trauma in the home and community or the effects of microaggressions in predominantly White spaces. Even more rare is the recognition of the role of race-based historical and intergenerational trauma, the effects of which can be passed down psychologically, behaviorally, and epigenetically. Historical and intergenerational trauma is immeasurably coursing through the veins of African Americans—atrocities such as racism, enslavement, and prejudice bring a loss of dignity that can rip through the soul.

Behavioral health providers are too frequently unaware of the historical and intergenerational trauma of the racialized populations they aim to help. With unrecognized and unacknowledged trauma, any other intervention could be aimed at the wrong target. Providers can easily overlook the ways that trauma effects have been transferred across generations for African Americans because history books have typically not revealed the whole story.

Intergenerational trauma responses may be transmitted through parenting behaviors and other interpersonal mechanisms. Behaviors as seemingly benign as not wanting to let go of a child's hand in a park, fear of dogs, wariness about traveling away from home, startle responses to certain stimuli, intense anger, or harsh discipline for minor infractions are all examples of people acting exactly as their ancestral history has wired them to.

Children can feel this anxiety even if they cannot understand it. In this way, trauma is communicated to the next generation. Those who are most susceptible to trauma and have the greatest trouble overcoming it have not only suffered their own trauma, but also come from a family in which their parents, and frequently their parents' parents, experienced trauma as well.

Understanding, identifying, and responding to the impacts of all forms of trauma is at the heart of the framework and organizational structure of trauma-informed care. Research highlights the necessity of including epigenetic effects in our increasing comprehension of how posttraumatic effects may be passed between generations.[26] Trauma-informed care helps clients regain a sense of control and empowerment while also prioritizing their physical, psychological, and emotional safety and the safety of the caregivers who assist them.[27]

Counselors must be able to look at a client and see. Listen to a client and hear. Sit with today's client and feel the intergenerational emotional and physical pain of yesterday's ancestor. Connect with a client and comprehend the visible and invisible trauma. Then celebrate the intergenerational survival: down through the years and still through the tears.

NOTES

1. James Weldon Johnson and J. Rosamond Johnson, "Lift Every Voice and Sing," (New York: E.B. Marks Music Co., 1921), https://www.loc.gov/resource/muslcdb .muslcdb-89751755/?st=gallery.

2. Faith Karimi and A.J. Willingham, "What Makes 'Lift Every Voice and Sing' so Iconic," CNN.com, September 10, 2020, https://www.cnn.com/interactive/2020/09/us/ lift-every-voice-and-sing-trnd.

3. Jennifer Mullan-Gonzalez, "Slavery and the Intergenerational Transmission of Trauma in Inner City African American Male Youth: A Model Program—from the Cotton Fields to the Concrete Jungle" (PhD diss., California Institute of Integral Studies, 2012).

4. SAMHSA's Trauma and Justice Strategic Initiative, "SAMHSA's Concept of Trauma," *SAMHSA's Concept of Trauma and Guidance for Trauma-Informed Approach* (July 2014): 7, https://ncsacw.acf.hhs.gov/userfiles/files/SAMHSA_Trauma.pdf.

5. Melanie Randall and Lori Haskell, "Trauma-Informed Approaches to Law: Why Restorative Justice Must Understand Trauma and Psychological Coping," *The Dalhousie Law Journal* 26 (2013): 501–33, https://ssrn.com/abstract=2424597.

6. Coral Muskett, "Trauma-Informed Care in Inpatient Mental Health Settings: A Review of the Literature," International Journal of Mental Health Nursing 23, no. 1 (2013): 51–59, https://doi.org/10.1111/inm.12012.

7. SAMHSA, *Trauma-Informed Care in Behavioral Health Services: TIP* 57 (March 2014), https://store.samhsa.gov/sites/default/files/d7/priv/sma14-4816.pdf.

8. *Merriam-Webster,* s.v. "trauma (*n.*),"https://www.merriam-webster.com/dictionary/ trauma.

9. Linda O'Neill et al., "Hidden Burdens: A Review of Intergenerational, Historical and Complex Trauma, Implications for Indigenous Families," *Journal of Child & Adolescent Trauma* 11, no. 2 (2016): 173–86, https://doi.org/10.1007/s40653-016-0117-9.

10. Maria Yellow Horse Brave Heart, "The Historical Trauma Response among Natives and Its Relationship with Substance Abuse: A Lakota Illustration," Journal of Psychoactive Drugs 35, no. 1 (2003): 7–13, https://doi.org/10.1080/02791072.2003.10399988.

11. Sue Coyle, "Intergenerational Trauma: Legacies of Loss," *Social Work Today* 14, no. 3 (May/June 2014): 18.

12. John J. Sigal, Vincenzo F. Dinicola, and Michael Buonvino, "Grandchildren of Survivors: Can Negative Effects of Prolonged Exposure to Excessive Stress Be Observed Two Generations Later?," *The Canadian Journal of Psychiatry* 33, no. 3 (1988): 207–12, https://doi.org/10.1177/070674378803300309.

13. Dora L. Costa, Noelle Yetter, and Heather DeSomer, "Intergenerational Transmission of Paternal Trauma among US Civil War Ex-Pows," *Proceedings of the National Academy of Sciences* 115, no. 44 (October 15, 2018): 11215–20, https://doi.org/10.1073/pnas.1803630115.

14. Rachel Yehuda et al., "Transgenerational Effects of Posttraumatic Stress Disorder in Babies of Mothers Exposed to the World Trade Center Attacks during Pregnancy," *The Journal of Clinical Endocrinology & Metabolism* 90, no. 7 (July 2005): 4115–8, https://doi.org/10.1210/jc.2005-0550.

15. Rachel Yehuda et al., "Holocaust Exposure Induced Intergenerational Effects on FKBP5 Methylation," *Biological Psychiatry* 80, no. 5 (August 12, 2015): 372–80, https://doi.org/10.1016/j.biopsych.2015.08.005.

16. Joy DeGruy Leary, *Post Traumatic Slave Syndrome: America's Legacy of Enduring Injury and Healing* (Portland, OR: Joy DeGruy Publications Inc., 2017), 48.

17. Nancy Boyd-Franklin, *Black Families in Therapy: Understanding the African American Experience*, 2nd ed. (New York, NY: Guilford Press, 2003), 8.

18. Phil Leask, "Losing Trust in the World: Humiliation and Its Consequences," Psychodynamic Practice 19, no. 2 (February 2013): 131, https://doi.org/10.1080/14753634.2013.778485.

19. Leask, "Losing Trust in the World," 132.

20. Sue Grand, "Skin Memories: On Race, Love and Loss," *Psychoanalysis, Culture &Amp; Society* 19, no. 3 (2014): 232–49, https://doi.org/10.1057/pcs.2014.24.

21. Saidiya Hartman, *Scenes of Subjection: Terror, Slavery, and Self-Making in Nineteenth Century America* (New York: Oxford University Press, 1997).

22. bell hooks, *Salvation: Black People and Love*, (New York, NY: Harper Collins / William Morrow Paperbacks, 2001).

23. Equal Justice Initiative, "Lynching in America: Confronting the Legacy of Racial Terror," accessed March 27, 2023, https://lynchinginamerica.eji.org/report.

24. Equal Justice Initiative, "Lynching in America."

25. Karina Margit Erdelyi, "Can Trauma Be Passed down from One Generation to the Next?" August 31, 2021, https://www.psycom.net/trauma/epigenetics-trauma.

26. Yehuda et al., "Transgenerational Effects."

27. Audria Greenwald, Amber Kelly, and Listy Thomas, "Trauma-Informed Care in the Emergency Department: Concepts and Recommendations for Integrating Practices into Emergency Medicine," Medical Education Online 28, no. 1 (February 17, 2023), https://doi.org/10.1080/10872981.2023.2178366.

The Emotional Weight of Carrying the Historical Presumption of Guilt

Nothing in the world is easier in the United States than to accuse a Black man of crime.

—*W. E. B. Du Bois*

RACIALIZATION AND CRIMINALIZATION IN THE UNITED STATES ARE two sides of the same coin.[1] Writing about mid-century Black criminality in crime fiction, author and university professor Theodore Martin draws attention to the pervasive cultural transmission of stereotypes about Black crime and criminality. In twentieth-century literature, Martin states, "crime was about race."[2]

The socio-political climate of the Civil Rights Movement demanded a change in the landscape of racial equity discussions. Jim Crow laws that had blatantly criminalized the everyday activities of Black people were overturned. Nonetheless, the condemnation of Blackness was still necessary for the established social hierarchy to continue.

THE NECESSITY OF BLACK GUILT

To retain the social hierarchy, it became crucial to continue equating Blackness with danger, thereby justifying the argument that Black people do not fit into the civility of American society. News reports of urban crime were—and often still are—subtly described with greater alarm than those of white-collar or suburban crime. Mainstream media perpetuated the stereotype of Black people as aggressive, criminal, and antagonistic. In news broadcasts, film, and television, the media disproportionately features Black people in situations where they are being physically restrained by law enforcement.

Through conscious and unconscious biases, Black criminalization perpetuated notions of Black inferiority, devaluing Black lives and invalidating Black productivity. Martin notes that "at a moment when crime and race were publicly bound together, crime fiction could not avoid the uncomfortable yet implacable fact that being Black in the U.S. was often synonymous with being seen as a criminal."[3]

This criminality became a common discourse, explained by racists as a problematic result of African American freedom and explained by African Americans and their allies as being a consequence of poverty. The greatest problem was that both sides of the argument accepted the myth of Black crime as a fact. Both factions bought into the problem of Black crime without debate. The debate was centered around the cause and the solution, rather than the widespread misperception of Blackness as criminality.[4]

Crime became a euphemism for Blackness. When people spoke of a "high crime area" it was a synonym for a Black neighborhood. The same was true when people mentioned a "bad part of town." While few White parents would say they have had a racial socialization conversation with their children in the way that African American and other Black parents have "the race talk" with their children, White parents actually do have such a conversation every time they tell their children to stay away from "bad" neighborhoods. By teaching their children that it's not safe and that they should be careful or take an alternate route to avoid the area, they can imply that the Black people who dwell or work in the area are not safe associations, planting seeds of suspicion and mistrust.

Bryan Stevenson, Director of the Equal Justice Initiative, speaks out about America's history of race-based guilt presumptions: "People of color have to cope with being watched and followed in stores and neighborhoods that are not their own. Being suspected, feared, and monitored at all times is frustrating and exhausting. In the criminal justice system, it is terrifying."[5] When law enforcement officials, prosecutors, courts, or anyone else incorrectly assumes that someone is guilty, lives are ruined, and horrifying injustices can occur.

The Weight of Black Guilt Starts Young

The emotional weight of carrying the historical presumptions of criminality and guilt falls on the shoulders of *all* Black people, young and old alike. This criminalization often begins in childhood, where studies show that African American and other Black children are subject to subtle dehumanization, harsher consequences because of age over-estimation, and greater culpability compared to their non-Black peers.[6]

Black boys as young as ten years old and Black girls as young as five years old are seen as less innocent, less in need of protection, and more adult than their White peers, and thus they are treated not as children but as mature adults deserving harsher punishment. They are assumed to be fully responsible for their actions and therefore experience harsh discipline for age-normative mistakes that could be addressed with restorative and non-punitive approaches.

The normal childlike behavior of their youthfulness is more often judged to be intentional and malicious rather than seen as simple immature decision-making. This phenomenon is known as "adultification" and it is part of a false narrative that the mistakes of a Black youth are actually intentional and therefore worthy of severe punishment. The presumption of guilt overrides any notion of an innocent, childlike mistake.[7] This issue has also been a factor in parenting: Black parenting styles are often more focused on addressing the outcome of behavior and less directed at assuming the innocence of a child's intent. Black children are then left to deal with assumptions of wrongdoing in both the home and in the community.

One important takeaway of the research associated with this pattern is the emphasis on the concept of innocence as an essential component of childhood. This innocence is more often assumed for White children than for Black children, giving White children better safeguards, whereas Black children are not as readily given a pass for any adolescent misdeeds.[8] Estimations of maturity and the resulting dismissal of innocence for Black children has a dehumanizing effect, especially given the fact that children are usually seen as the most vulnerable members of society and are afforded universal and mandated protections as such.

Research shows that Black children and adults were regarded as being much less innocent than White children and adults, or children and adults in general, for every age group beyond the age of nine. No variations in judgments of innocence between Whites and other people were found, either within an age group or overall.[9]

> Black innocence is hard to prove when Black guilt has already been assumed.

Children were seen as equally innocent from ages zero to nine regardless of race. However, by age ten, judgments of children's innocence started to differ. Starting at age ten, Black/African American children were thought of as considerably more culpable and less innocent than other children their age. In fact, the perceived level of innocence of ten- to thirteen-year-old Black children was seen as equivalent to that of fourteen- to seventeen-year-old non-Black children. Further, the perceived innocence of fourteen- to seventeen-year-old Black children was equivalent to the perceived innocence of eighteen- to twenty-one-year-old non-Black adults.[10]

This points to an innocence gap in which African American and other Black children have adult-like culpability prematurely put upon them. As children, they learn to carry a presumption of guilt. People tend to look disapprovingly at their age-normative behavior and assume that "they should know better!" Meanwhile, non-Black children are more likely to be ascribed the level of innocence they deserve for their age. We see dire repercussions of this innocence gap in mental health effects, education and academic problems, and criminal justice consequences.

Black children carry this age-inappropriate weight emotionally. With it come negative perceptions and expectations. Black children shoulder the burden of *being* no different but knowing that they are being *treated* differently than their non-Black peers, simply because of how people perceive them.

The Biopsychosocial Effects of the Guilt Burden

The weight of intolerance and exclusion is a heavy burden for people of any age. At all points in their lives, Black people are asked if they belong where they are. This issue of belonging can surface as early as kindergarten and persist throughout a person's education and development. It comes up when Black youngsters go shopping and are followed by store security; when they move to a new community and find cold-shouldered neighbors; when they go to a new school and are ignored during recess; when they ride their bikes and are met with distrusting looks; when they are frisked or assaulted simply for walking down the street; or when law enforcement or security officers are called in objection to their presence in places where they have a right to be. Proving that they belong there— as themselves—is a constant, weighty, mental and emotional labor. Yet, that labor can become such a part of life that they do not even recognize the fatigue or the burden at a conscious level.

Educational and Academic Problems

Black students walk through the classroom door carrying a burden of suspicion, expectations of lower achievement, and anticipated behavior problems (e.g., criminality). Why? Because teachers and administrators are not immune to the internalization of racialized messages and media images. Young Black children, even preschoolers, are often stereotyped as being violent, angry, or threatening at school. It is because of these stereotypes that they are disproportionately subjected to harsh disciplinary measures such as suspension or expulsion even when their behaviors are age normative.

Empirical research suggests that teachers may not always have the same academic expectations for Black pupils as they have for other students. Prejudices against racialized students include assumptions that they are less focused, less intelligent, and less likely to continue their education after high school. Early academic success has a significant impact on a child's sense of self-worth and the formation of a positive self-image in which they perceive themselves as intellectually competent, but racialized students are prone to seeing messages of inadequacy and hearing reasons to question their success.

Criminal Justice Consequences

The overrepresentation of Black Americans in the criminal justice system is a highly researched and well-documented fact. Research from the Brooklyn-based Vera Institute of Justice provides some staggering statistics. Representing roughly 13 percent of the US male population, Black men are approximately 35 percent of the prison population.[11] Data from The Sentencing Project shows highly disproportionate imprisonment rates for Black women as well. In 2021, the imprisonment rate for Black women was 62 per 100,000. That rate is 1.6 times the rate of imprisonment for White women at 38 per 100,000.[12]

A National Research Council report found that disparities in Black incarceration were caused by harsher legislation and the war on drugs, in addition to "small but systematic racial differences in case processing." Blacks, for example, had a higher likelihood of being imprisoned before going to trial, faring worse in plea deals that may have kept them out of jail, being arrested and charged with drug crimes that have stiff mandatory penalties, or receiving the death penalty.[13] Nearly half (48.3 percent) of life and virtual life-sentenced individuals are African American.[14]

COUNSELOR SELF-AWARENESS

Counselors cannot afford to be ill-equipped for recognizing and responding to clients who carry the emotional weight of the historical presumption of guilt. Systemic double standards positioned White people as innocent until proven guilty and Black people as guilty until proven innocent. This can be true in communities, schools, courtrooms, and retail stores, or while walking down the street or driving down a highway. Black innocence is hard to prove when Black guilt has already been assumed. But innocence and guilt are not limited to the criminal justice system. All concerns, events, relationships, and systemic practices that affect Black people are quietly infused with disparities or disadvantages. When counselors allow themselves to be mindful of the burden of suspicion that any

Black client may experience on any given day, they can better listen for racial meaning within their clients' experiences.

When working with children and teens, a counselor must use age-appropriate interventions and have similarly adjusted expectations. Counselors can easily miss their own tendency toward overestimation of a child's age or over-assessment of a young person's culpability. Those are psychosocial patterns that can influence anyone, including the most seasoned, well-intentioned counselors.

Counselors might easily overlook the inherent invalidating messages of some of our most commonly used theories and interventions. Counseling techniques and interventions that focus on anger management and behavior modification without accurate empathy and client advocacy can perpetuate the burden of "getting it right" or the message that a young client "should know better."

Counselors must engage in introspective inquiry to assess their biases and ask themselves the hard questions:

- Do I have equitable expectations of all clients?
- Do I recognize when a client's attempt at self-advocacy is pathologized, met with disfavor, or punished by other individuals and systems in their life?
- Am I invalidating a client's experience with interventions aimed at changing the client rather than the biased system?
- Am I unfairly pathologizing experiences that need to be normalized?
- Do my biases cause me to unjustly normalize client experiences that should not be normalized?
- Have I benefited from, or participated in, the expectation that Black people need to prove that they belong in spaces where I didn't expect to see them?
- Are there ways in which I dismiss, devalue, or deny a client's lived reality?
- Am I overestimating a young Black client's culpability?

- Do I dehumanize a client with adultification or denial of their childhood innocence? In other words, am I quick to think, *They're old enough to know better*?

One of the counseling profession's core values is "honoring diversity and embracing a multicultural approach in support of the worth, dignity, potential, and uniqueness of people within their social and cultural contexts."[15] May we support that dignity in ways that demand that society unburden those who carry any historical presumption of guilt.

NOTES

1. Theodore Martin, "Crime Fiction and Black Criminality," *American Literary History* 30, no. 4 (October 17, 2018): 703–29, https://doi.org/10.1093/alh/ajy037.

2. Martin, "Crime Fiction."

3. Martin, "Crime Fiction."

4. Martin, "Crime Fiction."

5. Equal Justice Initiative, "The Presumption of Guilt," July 11, 2022, https://eji.org/issues/presumption-of-guilt.

6. Phillip Atiba Goff et al., "The Essence of Innocence: Consequences of Dehumanizing Black Children," *Journal of Personality and Social Psychology* 106, no. 4 (April 2014): 526–45, https://doi.org/10.1037/a0035663; Adrienne Green, "How Black Girls Aren't Presumed to Be Innocent," *The Atlantic*, June 29, 2017, https://www.theatlantic.com/politics/archive/2017/06/black-girls-innocence-georgetown/532050.

7. Green, "How Black Girls."

8. Green, "How Black Girls."

9. Goff, et al., "The Essence of Innocence."

10. Goff, et al., "The Essence of Innocence."

11. Elizabeth Kai Hinton, LeShae Henderson, and Cindy Reed, "An Unjust Burden," Vera.org, Vera Institute of Justice, May 2018, https://www.vera.org/publications/for-the-record-unjust-burden.

12. Nikki Monazzam and Kristen Budd, "Incarcerated Women and Girls," The Sentencing Project, April 3, 2023, https://www.sentencingproject.org/fact-sheet/incarcerated-women-and-girls.

13. National Research Council, *The Growth of Incarceration in the United States: Exploring Causes and Consequences* (Washington, DC: The National Academies Press, 2014), https://doi.org/10.17226/18613.

14. Ashley Nellis, "America's Increasing Use of Life and Long-Term Sentences," *The Sentencing Project*, November 2, 2022, https://www.sentencingproject.org/reports/still-life-americaos-increasing-use-of-life-and-long-term-sentences.

15. American Counseling Association, *2014 ACA Code of Ethics Preamble—American Counseling Association*, https://www.counseling.org/resources/aca-code-of-ethics.pdf.

Part III

Overlooked Clinical Bias

CHAPTER 6

The Problem of Counselor Colorblindness

Racism is a complex and interconnected system that adapts to challenges over time. Colorblind ideology was a very effective adaptation to the challenges of the Civil Rights Era. Colorblind ideology allows society to deny the reality of racism in the face of its persistence, while making it more difficult to challenge than when it was openly espoused.

—ROBIN DiANGELO

The notion of a colorblind society, in which all people are regarded as belonging to the "human race," is a popular view in racial discourse. Such colorblindness, however, carries dissimilar meanings for racialized groups than for Whites. For African Americans and others who identify as Black, colorblindness works *against* their interests. Colorblindness acknowledges that everyone is *created* equal but overlooks the fact that everyone has not been *treated* equally. Every client has the same inherent human dignity, but not every client has lived without the fear of their dignity being denied.

If "I don't see color" is meant to imply that "I appreciate and treat all individuals equally," then it is undoubtedly an admirable sentiment. For counseling professionals, however, this creates a problem because the ethics of our profession demand that we directly attend to diversity.

Although the road of colorblindness is paved with good intentions, it allows an insidious denial of the experiential differences of racialized groups. The invalidating nature of colorblindness makes it a type of microaggression known as *microinvalidation*.

But why does a person feel the need to be colorblind to racial diversity? If unacknowledged diversity feels noble or unbiased, should that be challenged? Has a counselor touting colorblindness considered that racial acknowledgment does not have to automatically carry the implication of racial bias? These are difficult questions, but leaving them unanswered can allow diversity barriers to loom within your clinical practice.

As long as a person does not see race, they need not address the discriminatory racial system in which we live.

In 2016, the American Psychological Association published a prolific edited volume titled, "The Myth of Racial Colorblindness."[1] In chapter three, James M. Jones draws attention to the fact that from a medical stance, colorblindness by definition is a deficiency that prevents people from clearly distinguishing a full spectrum of colors. Rhetorically, Jones asks, "But if color blindness is a deficiency, why is it lauded as a virtue of character when it comes to perceiving racial differences?"[2] Jones suggests that racial colorblindness consists of four beliefs:

> (a) skin color is superficial and irrelevant to the quality of a person's character, ability, or worthiness; (b) in a merit-based society, skin color is irrelevant to merit judgments and calculations of fairness; (c) a corollary of (b)—judgments of merit and fairness are flawed if race is included in their calculation; and (d) ignoring skin color when interacting with people is the best way to avoid racial discrimination.[3]

Jones aptly explains that these beliefs actually perpetuate racial hierarchy, relieve the holders of any responsibility, and allow biases to go without scrutiny.[4]

When I teach diversity courses, I regularly hear well-meaning White counselors and students proudly boast, "I don't see race. I don't see color. I was taught to be colorblind." The colorblind approach to racial diversity sounds noble, but at its core represents an ideology of avoidance—it serves as an unwitting euphemism for "There is nothing to talk about." But European settlers in North America created a racial identity system for the United States that is older than the country itself. A colorblind approach to race gives people the opportunity to avoid talking about the devastation and current reality of that system. So, we *must* talk about it!

What I Am About to Say

"What I'm about to say to you has nothing to do with race." Would a White supervisor use that as a disclaimer in a corrective action conversation with a White employee? Does a White parent respond to their White child's playground fight with another White child by saying, "I'm so sorry; I try to teach them to be colorblind"?

Would a White supervisor or parent use such statements with a Black person? It's certainly possible, because a colorblind stance actually says, "I do see the color of your skin, but let's not talk about it. I don't want you to think I'm being prejudiced."

Are anti-discrimination and pro-diversity two sides of the same proverbial coin? The concept of colorblindness implies an anti-discriminatory approach to race relations. However, rather than boosting equity, colorblindness minimizes the goodness in diversity and promotes a sameness that further strips or devalues the identity of historically marginalized races and ethnicities. Therein lies the danger for a counselor—colorblindness is individualistic and self-protective, causing systemic issues to be blurred and both race *and* the reality of injustices to be dismissed. As long as a person does not see race, they need not address the discriminatory racial system in which we live.

Colorblindness *appears* to reflect pro-diversity beliefs, but actually diminishes diversity. In turn, it gives license for cultural insensitivity to the lived reality of African Americans and other Black people in America. With a true pro-diversity mindset, we do pay attention to race and other elements of diversity so that the client has the necessary space to address the issues and emotions of their lived reality. Pro-diversity practice acknowledges both race and the discriminatory systems that keep racially minoritized communities disempowered.

A person says they do not see color instead of truthfully acknowledging their concern: "I assume that talking about race makes me a racist because the conversations I hear about race *are* often racist." Clearly, race is not unseen in America, and race must no longer be sidelined in the counselor–client interaction.

THE NEED FOR COLOR CONSCIOUSNESS

Culturally responsive color consciousness, or race consciousness, in counseling is the capacity to be aware of race, race-based trauma, and the effects of race in clients' lives. Race consciousness steps away from the all-or-nothing polarity of prejudicial race responses (intentional racism) or racial unresponsiveness (unintentional racism). Counselors with appropriate color consciousness invite conversations about race and injustice to come from the background to the foreground of their clinical work. Race-conscious counselors actively support racial justice and racial equity as a central part of their work.

In American culture, race identities can be perceived as both visible and invisible. In the same moment, those lives are both valued and devalued. Their experiences are simultaneously relevant and irrelevant. Their movement is at once liberated and constrained. Clients may encounter this and be unable to articulate the contradiction and incongruence. For this reason, counselors must purposefully move dialogues about race and injustice to the forefront of the counselor–client dialogue. As a fundamental aspect of their profession, race-conscious counselors advocate for racial justice and equality.

Multiple researchers in the field of behavioral health consider colorblindness to be a means of evading America's racial and power disparities. That which we avoid cannot be honored. We cannot respect something we deny. A colorblind racial ideology is unethical from this point of view, while a race-aware philosophy leaves the door open for ethical conduct.

When a counselor uses a colorblind racial ideology in therapy, the risk of doing harm is palpable. A crucial aspect of the client's story is ignored and undervalued when a counselor interacts with a client without understanding the realities of race and culture. When the unique context of BIPOC life is not understood, the counselor will engage in generic therapies that overlook key aspects of Black life in America. When racial discrimination and power imbalances are downplayed, the colorblind person can hold the victim responsible for the injustices and maltreatment they face. Colorblindness says that "Anyone can get ahead in this country if they are willing to work hard" or "The American dream is available to anyone!" Colorblindness overlooks ways in which members of racialized groups are often positioned outside of institutional and systemic structures that are accessible to others, but are simultaneously blamed for not holding the key that unlocks the doors.

HOW SHIFT HAPPENS

Oh, how gratifying when a client adjusts a lens and sees their situation from a new perspective. This is also a task for counselors who choose to shift from a colorblind worldview into a color-conscious vision of humanity. This kind of a counselor shift can significantly increase the counselor's effectiveness.

Out of the Shadows

First, the topic of race needs to come out of the shadows. A counselor must overcome any fear of introducing race-related content during a session with clients. When race and culture are ignored in the therapeutic discourse, culture becomes incidental and is only sometimes mentioned. When counselors bring the identity elements of race and culture to the foreground, both the client and the counselor can explore how these identities interact with the presenting concerns of therapy. Otherwise, we are silently saying, "I know you are Black, but let's separate that from your presenting concern of parenting teenagers or your concerns about getting a promotion at work, or healing your marriage, or managing your anxiety. Surely there are no racial nuances to *those* problems!" Sounds silly, right? Of course, there are likely to be racial elements to any of those concerns for a client who identifies as Black or African American!

Be open to hearing about the racial experiences and concerns of Black clients. What's their story of race? Were they pioneers in integrating a community, a school, or a place of worship? If so, how did that impact them? Was trauma involved in those events? Are there other sources of race-related trauma, such as being victimized by a person of another race, or losing a loved one in a race-related incident? What additional hurdles did they, their parents, or their grandparents overcome? There are many approaches for gleaning this important information. If you need some time to progressively move into conversational content naturally, you can start by adding racial trauma questions to the trauma background section of the intake or client information form.

Unpack Your Own Story

Second, explore your own history of race relations and encounters. Write your race narrative as a personal project. Everyone's experience with race and interracial encounters is distinct. The exercise of writing a race narrative allows the counselor to consider how race-related events have impacted their identity, perceptions, emotional reactions, behavior, and interpersonal connections. The race narrative questions listed below are designed to help counselors examine what they have learned about race and what they have done with race-related situations. This assists counselors in bringing their racial story to the foreground. Eventually, counselors may also choose to incorporate race narrative segments with client interventions.

Example Race Narrative Questions

1. How do you self-describe racially? Ethnically? Has that changed over time?

2. When growing up, how did your family of origin self-describe racially and ethnically?

3. Do you have immediate or extended family members who self-describe as biracial or multiracial? If so, how have you experienced your relationship with them?

4. Do you see yourself as marginalized or privileged? When responding, please consider whether you have race privilege, economic privilege, both, or neither.

5. What was your age and first impression the first time you saw or met a person of another race?

6. What roles have people of other races had in your life (e.g., friend, childhood caregiver, housekeeper, teacher, professional peer, professional supervisor, religious leader)?

7. Is there a person of another race who has been positively influential in your life? What kind of influence did they have?

8. Have you ever been personally victimized by a person of another race? If so, what effect did that have on your perspectives on race?

9. What were the implicit or explicit messages you took in growing up about *your* race? About *other* races?

10. To what extent have you crossed "racial lines" (e.g., school integration or neighborhood integration) voluntarily or involuntarily. How would you describe that experience?

11. Have you ever confronted someone about statements or behaviors that you believed to be racist, segregationist, racially inflammatory, discriminatory, or racially unjust? What was that experience like?

12. What stereotypes, prejudices, or forms of discrimination do you think you may have personally subscribed to over the years?

13. What might it cost you professionally, socially, relationally, or financially to position yourself differently in controversial race-related conversations?

14. To what extent has your racial identity in America benefited you or limited you?

15. How old were you when you first realized that the original color of adhesive bandages was not designed with all skin tones in mind? What (other) norms or standards have you overlooked?

A counselor's racial narrative has power because it prompts the counselor to acknowledge the presence and sources of their presumptions and prejudices. This kind of introspection and contemplation are necessary for the ethical practice of counseling.

Destigmatize Race

Third, commit to "seeing" color without bias in racialized clients. Ask yourself if you have been exposed to bias that sees racialized groups as "marked" people or their race as a source of shame and embarrassment. Anti-racist counselors see no shame in another person's ancestry, whether African, Asian, Hispanic, Indigenous, or another heritage. Colorblindness suggests that there is either something to be ignored, some disadvantage or point of shame we should not discuss, or a heritage not worthy of recognition. Instead, counselors must see the person's heritage as a strength—and tell them that's what you see! When counselors avoid confronting historical racial issues and power differentials, they can easily blame the victim for the hardships they face.

See the Story

Lastly, appreciate the client's racial and cultural story. It is not bad to respectfully acknowledge someone's race. It's not a bad thing to acknowledge your own race. When you look at the face of a racialized person, see the history behind every wrinkle. See the remnants of ancestral trauma. See the scars of the intergenerational battles in a world that has tried to marginalize them. See their resilience. See them. Respect them. See the residual effects of slavery. See the descendants of abolitionists. See them overcoming myths and stereotypes. Join them in valuing their culture in a world that devalues it and tries to make it invisible. See the legacy of survival they have inherited. Mourn with them! Celebrate with them! Let them know you respect and meet them in whatever space they find themselves.

NOTES

1. Helen A. Neville, Miguel E. Gallardo, and Derald Wing Sue, eds., *The Myth of Racial Color Blindness: Manifestations, Dynamics, and Impact* (Washington, DC: American Psychological Association, 2016).

2. James M. Jones, "The Color-Blind Racial Approach—Does Race Really Matter?," in *The Myth of Racial Color Blindness: Manifestations, Dynamics, and Impact*, ed. Helen A.

Neville, Miguel E. Gallardo, and Derald Wing Sue (Washington, DC: American Psychological Association, 2016): 39–52.

3. Jones, "The Color-Blind Racial Approach."

4. Jones, "The Color-Blind Racial Approach."

CHAPTER 7

Marginalized vs. Privileged Expectations and Assumptions in Counseling

Privilege is not something I take and which therefore have the option of not taking.
It is something that society gives me, and unless I change the institutions which give it to me,
they will continue to give it, and I will continue to have it,
however noble and equalitarian my intentions.

—HARRY BROD

CLASSISM IS A FACT OF LIFE IN THE UNITED STATES AND AROUND THE world. The distinction between "the haves and the have-nots" is a stubborn stain on any nation or society. In the United States, the "American dream" of owning a home and a car (or maybe two or three), the status afforded by college degrees, and the luxuries of financial wealth suggest that privilege includes the freedom of choice. It includes power. It includes opportunity. Our society's "measures of success" could also be called "indicators of economic privilege."

When I reference privilege, I am referencing advantageous social positions, whether achieved or ascribed. White privilege, or race privilege, is in the category of ascribed privilege, which means it is assigned by society. Economic privilege is in the category of achieved privilege and is based on financial advantage.

I have a friend: middle-aged, White, Christian, heterosexual, male. He sat across from me as we spoke about the social, cultural, political, and economic events of that year. It was 2016 just a few weeks after the end of a biting and bitter presidential campaign and election. He held a community leadership position that carried great respect in our town. With him, I was always able to talk about difficult things—with mutual respect—and he used to say that I helped him become a better leader. We shared many of the same beliefs and values.

On this particular day, I spoke frankly about my concerns amid the events of that time. I felt heard, seen, and understood—that is, until we began talking about White privilege. He quickly came to his own rescue, as if he sensed danger on the horizon. "I'm not privileged," he said. "I grew up in a poor rural area. Times were hard for us and there was nothing about my life that even remotely looked privileged." He asked me not to include him when I used the words "White privilege."

That was not the only time I have heard someone hold steadfastly to denying their privilege. Every time, it has been because they did not make a distinction between White privilege and economic privilege. The two can occur together, but that is not always the case. An individual can self-identify with any race or ethnicity and have some degree of economic privilege. Even though Black and other racialized groups are underrepresented in the ranks of American wealth, economic privilege is not totally race dependent. White privilege, however, is the privilege of not having to be concerned about factors related to a racialized life.

Figure 7.1 depicts the experiences of White and BIPOC privilege and marginalization. A person can be Black or White *with* economic privilege. A person can be Black or White *without* the advantage of economic privilege. However, a person *cannot* be Black and have White privilege in our society. And if they are White, they automatically have White privilege.

The **Protected** lifestyle comes with freedom and opportunities. With both economic privilege and race privilege, the key distinguishing factor is the degree of choice that is available and the ability to move through life without thinking about economic survival or race-based discrimination. This experience comes with the opportunity for financial stability,

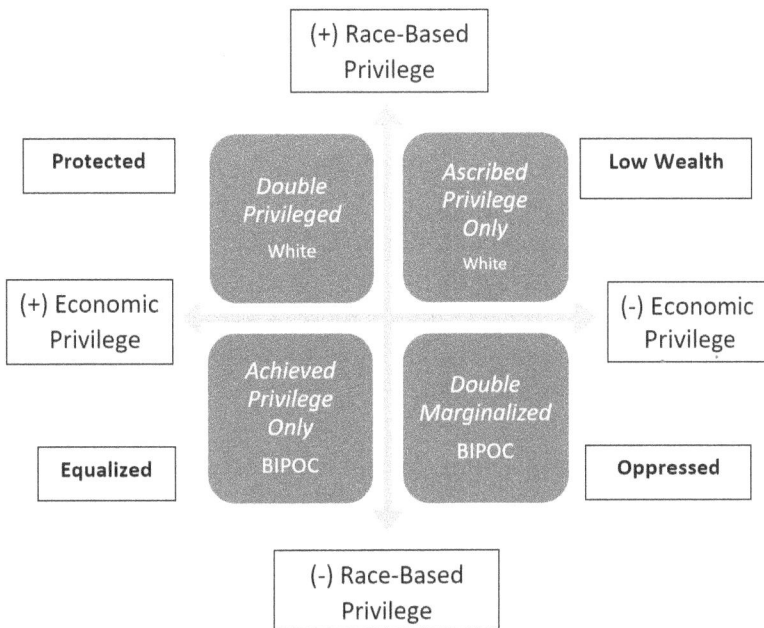

Figure 7.1 Collins Four Worldviews of Privilege.

building generational wealth, more choices of neighborhoods, better health care options, and more disposable income.

Those living an ***Equalized*** lifestyle may also have more choices and more opportunities for financial stability, economic mobility, better health care options, more disposable income, and other financially stabilizing factors. But this is not equality, and this group is not the same as the *Protected* group. The "equalized" experience represents the intersection of economic privilege and racial marginalization. Their economic privilege may grant them a level of prestige or influence within their own social circles, but in places where their economic privilege is not known, they are subject to the same risks and barriers as a person without economic privilege. In some White or racially mixed spaces where they are known, their achieved privilege can be an equalizer in *some* of their life experience. Therefore, while they have choices in many areas, they do not have the ability to move through life without concerns about race-based discrimination. They are racially marginalized by the larger society but economically privileged, thus potentially giving them some social capital, professional relationships, and financial resources to fight injustice and legal battles when they do arise. These can be equalizing factors in a society where equality does not exist.

The *Low Wealth* lifestyle affords fewer choices because of economic limitations. It is the early life experience of my friend who denied having any privilege. Those with this lifestyle benefit from White privilege, especially in places where they are not known, but they may find any type of privilege difficult to admit because of the absence of financial stability and economic mobility. Their economic frame of reference brings challenges in health care, education, and housing, causing feelings of economic disempowerment. Where economic privilege is lacking, many people with this experience view the maintenance of race privilege as crucial. This sounds paradoxical to the frequent denial of race privilege, but race may be the only capital that some *Low Wealth* people believe they have.

The *Oppressed* are Black, Indigenous, and People of Color (BIPOC) who have neither race privilege nor economic privilege. Their experiences in the depths of marginalization can feel inescapable, as they move through life with combined concerns about both race-based discrimination and economic survival. The circumstances of this group commonly call for greater advocacy and social justice interventions such as writing letters about inhumane conditions, securing referrals to human aid services, or advocating in schools or hospitals.

The ascribed statuses of race and ethnicity are generally seen as unchanging, unless a person decides to "pass" in society as another race or self-identify with another aspect of their ancestry. However, people can move between economic positions. Many people grow up in poverty but attain wealth later in life. Others may start out in life inheriting or attaining economic privilege but later lose that position or choose a different lifestyle.

Human nature is vexed with a degree of tunnel vision—a propensity to see situations from our own frame of reference.

A culturally sensitive counselor is cognizant of their own economic frame of reference in addition to that of their clients with different experiences. The values, choices, barriers, and problem-solving approaches of each position will vary. Human nature is vexed with a degree of tunnel vision—a propensity to see situations from our own frame of reference. Not only do we tend to see the problems of other people through our own lens, but we tend to cast a disparaging eye toward that which is different from our personal lived reality.

Much of America views privilege as normative. Those who lack economic privilege are stereotyped as lacking motivation, stupid, deserving of their fate, unable to rise above it, lazy, or unwilling to "pull themselves up by the bootstraps like 'everyone else' in this country."[1] Classist structures are always established and maintained by the privileged class. Omitted from the mainstream narrative is the paradoxical revelation that marginalized people are criticized for not faring well in a system *designed* to keep them from doing so.[2]

Cullen Hightower once wrote, "Only the poor can know all the disadvantages of poverty. Only the rich can know all the disadvantages of wealth."[3] Reflected in this statement is the reality that others, even counselors, who have had different life experiences are quite often oblivious to the challenges faced by economically disadvantaged communities. In fact, counselors from wealthier backgrounds may have trouble empathizing with people living in poverty. Counselors may struggle to grasp how poverty causes unstable living arrangements, poor health, difficulties with consistent attendance or punctuality for sessions, and a variety of other issues that are unfamiliar to those from more economically stable backgrounds.

Dougall and Schwartz found that therapists reacted differently to a client with a privileged versus a marginalized socioeconomic presentation in a therapy session. Their study examined how a client's socioeconomic presentation might impact the provider's countertransference reaction. They found that with an economically privileged client, countertransference was triggered, and the counselor experienced the client as coming from a place of dominance.[4] Ideally, a counselor's awareness and self-insight into their countertransference will prevent biased reactions to the client. Otherwise, a counselor is likely to violate any number of ethical principles.

This study and others found that socioeconomics can affect a counselor's clinical judgments about a client. Dougall and Schwartz highlighted that the client's problems were either over-pathologized or minimized based on the client's socioeconomic characteristics. Specifically, they found that negative clinical judgments caused therapists to rate the problems of economically privileged clients as milder, while the problems of marginalized clients were rated as more severe, despite only having ambiguous information about each client's presenting problems.[5]

IN-GROUP ECONOMIC BIAS

The Equalized—economically privileged—members of marginalized groups may harbor biases toward people of their own race or ethnicity based on their economic status. This happens as a result of the privileges and power differences conferred upon people by economics rather than race. Therefore, even if a person does not have racial privilege, their economic advantage may cause them to cast a wary eye toward members of their own race or ethnicity who are impoverished. This is an intra-racial form of "othering."

Meanwhile, a co-occurring dynamic is also possible. The Oppressed—doubly marginalized—may see the Equalized as selling out or "acting White." The acting White accusation is a counterattack to discredit economic privilege within Black experiences, and can be highly insulting to African American people who are attaining their educational, professional, or financial aspirations.

These dynamics create a dual strain for those who must simultaneously contend with interracial bias based on color and intraracial bias based on economics. Class bias—in either direction—within one's race can be highly demoralizing. Clients who experience this type of othering may be hesitant to express their sentiments to someone of a different race or socioeconomic position.

An Oppressed (doubly marginalized) person's response to this double alienation can show up in strong retorts: "They think they're better than everyone else," "She got her nose all up in the air," "He's stuck up!" or "They think they're too good for us!" Such sentiments offer a protective self-conceptualization to counter frame the denigrating effects of classism. This manner of reframing and counter-framing are common protective behaviors for the self-esteem of people who are made to feel different by classism, racism, or other types of prejudice.[6]

In 2021, Spates and Slatton examined factors that contribute to Black women's resilience. Interestingly, 45 percent of the participating women viewed social and economic privilege differently than the dominant culture. These women perceived their social location as a strength. They viewed White males as weaker and less capable of dealing with

Table 7.1 Collins's Counselor Self-Assessment of Class-Based Bias

1. How do I describe my current economic status? How is that like, or unlike, my family's economic position during my formative years?
2. What messages did I learn about people from social classes other than my own?
3. Do I see socioeconomic status as an element of the client's cultural diversity?
4. When I make a comparative list of diagnoses or problems that I ascribe to wealthy clients, how does that compare to the diagnoses and problems that I ascribe to low-income clients?
5. How do I feel when I am with economically privileged clients? How do I feel with clients who are less economically privileged? Do I recognize any countertransference in those interactions?
6. How can I be more sensitive to the challenges of economically disadvantaged people?
7. What are the systemic or institutional barriers to care faced by low-wealth and oppressed people in my community or my practice? What can I do to advocate for them?
8. How might my values and worldview impact the therapeutic process when I am working with someone from a different economic background?
9. Do I attempt to use treatment approaches or have assumptions that lack economic sensitivity or promote classism?
10. Do I regularly include the challenges of economic class in my case consultations or clinical supervision?
11. What message does my personal life convey about people in each of the four lifestyles presented in this section: Protected, Equalized, Low-Wealth, and Oppressed?
12. Is there an immersion experience I can engage in to increase my awareness of poverty's plight (e.g., living in a homeless shelter for thirty days)? Am I willing to do that?

adversity because they had an easy existence and had not acquired the resilience needed to withstand challenges.[7]

Culturally astute counselors are aware of the damage inflicted by classism within and between cultures. It is the obligation of the counselor to consider whether economic disparities are a contributing cause of the client's current issue. This is a matter of ethical conduct and advocacy for social justice. With a keen awareness of how systemic, institutional, interpersonal, and intrapersonal classism impacts their clients, counselors will be better positioned to serve their economically and socially underprivileged clients. Table 7.1 includes some reflection questions to help build counselors' self-awareness.

Therapists need to be conscious of how their personal economic history may color their perspectives and treatment of clients. Professionally, counselors owe it to people who have been oppressed by classism to practice cultural humility and sensitivity. Therapists should be prepared to address class bias head-on in their work with clients through acts of social justice and advocacy.

Classism is deeply embedded in American society, yet it does not receive the same level of attention as racism or sexism as a form of discrimination. Classism is an issue that transcends color, ethnicity, gender, age, sexual orientation, and many other cultural markers. Introspective counselors who take seriously the work of self-exploration will be more cognizant of class biases that may damage their therapeutic rapport and the treatment results of their clients.

NOTES

1. LaVerne Collins, "Fighting Classism," *Counseling Today* (September 2022): 14.

2. Collins, "Fighting Classism."

3. "Top 50 Cullen Hightower Quotes of All Time," Quotes.pub, accessed April 6, 2023, https://quotes.pub/cullen-hightower-quotes.

4. Jennifer L. Dougall and Robert C. Schwartz, "The Influence of Client Socioeconomic Status on Psychotherapists' Attributional Biases and Countertransference Reactions," *American Journal of Psychotherapy* 65, no. 3 (2011): 249–65, https://doi.org/10.1176/appi.psychotherapy.2011.65.3.249.

5. Dougall and Schwartz, "The Influence," 260.

6. Collins, "Fighting Classism."

7. Kamesha Spates and Brittany C Slatton, "Repertoire of Resilience: Black Women's Social Resistance to Suicide," *Social Problems* 70, no. 3 (August 2023): 650–64, https://doi.org/10.1093/socpro/spab072.

Chapter 8

Diagnostic Bias

Cultural incompetence of health care providers likely contributes to underdiagnosis and/or misdiagnosis of mental illness in BIPOC.
—*Mental Health America*

Underdiagnosed. Overdiagnosed. Misdiagnosed. Diagnostic errors for African American and other Black clients are both common and overlooked. Racial inequality in mental health care can be tied to several causative factors, but provider bias is among the most dangerous. It is a long-standing problem dating back to the use of psychiatry to justify Black inferiority and uphold the cruelties of slavery.

When enslaved people desired freedom and attempted to flee, they were diagnosed with "drapetomania," which is "a form of mania supposedly affecting slaves and manifested by an uncontrollable impulse to wander or run away from their White masters."[1] When slaves behaviorally resisted, they were diagnosed with "dysaesthesia aethiopica," another "mental illness" described as the cause of rascality and laziness among slaves.[2]

Both terms were coined and advanced by a physician named Dr. Samuel A. Cartwright.[3] When these behaviors were present, Cartwright proposed that the treatment was to cut off one or both of the person's big toes. Cartwright also advised slaveholders to regularly and mercilessly whip the enslaved until they understood their lower positionality in the world and changed their behavior. Cartwright practiced in several southern states and authored several papers addressing the "Diseases and Peculiarities of the Negro Race."[4] These contrived diagnoses are evidence that normalcy and psychopathology can be heavily influenced by economics, culture, and the personal values of the diagnostician.

In contemporary medicine, the problem of provider bias usually occurs at a more unconscious level, but it is still cause for great concern. Provider bias can contribute to inaccuracies in case conceptualizations and diagnostic impressions, resulting in poor treatment outcomes, early withdrawal from treatment, under- or overmedication of patients, and clinical interventions aimed at the wrong targets. In this chapter, we examine ways that under-, over-, and misdiagnosis commonly affect Black Americans. It is impossible to measure the frequency at which diagnostic errors occur in mental health care. However, we can look at the prevalence of disparities in key diagnostic categories and we can commit ourselves to self-awareness and systemic change.

I coined the term "biasnosis" to describe a diagnosis given when a counselor's unconscious bias influences their interpretation of clinical symptoms. Biasnosis is responsible for clinicians seeing and interpreting symptoms differently based on a client's race. Mental Health America (MHA) reports that Black men in particular are likely to be given incorrect psychiatric diagnoses that are especially severe, or less treatable.[5] The various research studies and cases presented in this chapter point to ways that bias can be involved in the diagnoses of schizophrenia, depression, eating disorders in adults, and learning/developmental disabilities, autism spectrum disorder, and other disorders in Black children.

THE OVERDIAGNOSIS OF SCHIZOPHRENIA

Schizophrenia is a mental disorder characterized by disruptions in thought processes, perceptions, emotional responsiveness, and social interactions.[6] According to the American Psychiatric Association's Diagnostic and Statistical Manual of Mental Disorders, fifth edition, text revision (*DSM-5-TR*), schizophrenia is an illness that must be diagnosed by exclusion, which means that its symptoms must not be explainable by another mental health disorder, such as a mood disorder.[7] Despite this criteria, Black people are substantially more likely than White people to be diagnosed with schizophrenia alone, even when a mood disorder is present, according to an MHA report.[8]

MHA found that clinicians tend to overemphasize the relevance of psychotic symptoms and overlook symptoms of major depression when treating Black clients, compared to when they are treating clients with other racial or ethnic backgrounds. As a result, Black men are four times more likely to be diagnosed with schizophrenia than White men.[9]

Jameson's Story

Jameson is a thirty-six-year-old Jamaican American male with a history of mild to moderate depression. He works as a massage therapist in an upscale day spa. His professional training in massage therapy gives him a good understanding of the human musculoskeletal system, so when Jameson injured his shoulder while playing basketball with his sons, he recognized that his severe pain could be an indication of a dislocated shoulder.

Jameson went to the hospital emergency room, but the attending physician refused to give him any pain medicine. She saw a Black man in physical discomfort and believed he was a medication-seeking drug addict. The doctor dismissed the severity of the shoulder pain even when Jameson explained that over-the-counter meds were not helping him, and the pain had not subsided in the forty-eight hours since the injury occurred. The doctor continued to minimize Jameson's account of his pain, saying, "A big Black guy like you can handle a little shoulder pain without popping pills."

Jameson became tearful and visibly annoyed at being stereotyped as a drug-seeker. With the pain worsening, he questioned the doctor, "Why are you doing this to me? What reason do you have?" The doctor's response was to "biasnose" Jameson with paranoid schizophrenia and flag him as med-seeking on his medical chart. She discharged him from the emergency room, saying there was nothing she could do for him. The next day at a different facility, Jameson was examined by an orthopedic specialist who confirmed that Jameson's shoulder was dislocated.

Black men are disproportionately diagnosed with schizophrenia because of provider bias in clinical judgment. The emergency room doctor had two biases operating in this case. She characterized Black men as drug abusers and she pathologized the Black man's self-advocacy efforts. Providers have a responsibility to listen to clients and not make biased assumptions, but too often, African American and other Black voices are unheard.

THE UNDERDIAGNOSIS OF EATING DISORDERS

Marcia is a twenty-five-year-old, never-married, cisgendered African American female. She recently moved to a new city and a new job, leaving behind her friends and family. She wanted a fresh start, so she decided to begin seeing a counselor about some long-standing issues. Marcia nervously opened up about her struggle with food restriction and compulsive exercise. She acknowledged that socially she covers up her insecurities with her jovial personality, but secretly she continually body-shames herself. Her self-hatred and fear were spiraling out of control. Marcia described obsessively and compulsively trying to manage every germ, every calorie, and every perceived risk. Marcia also described frequent moodiness and irritability.

Marcia had never shared her struggle with anyone before this. It felt like a relief to get it all out in the open. Marcia really wanted to get her eating disorder under control and learn to manage her obsessive-compulsive behavior. But every counseling appointment was a huge disappointment.

The first counselor listened to Marcia's extreme obsession about managing germs, calories, and death, and "biasnosed" Marcia with paranoid personality disorder. Another counselor "biasnosed" her eating disorder as adjustment disorder. A third counselor "biasnosed" her with bipolar disorder because of the moodiness she experienced (probably from just being undernourished.) They recommended antipsychotics and antidepressants for problems she did not have, while her OCD and eating disorder continued to worsen.

Marcia was not the skinny, delicate White girl that many mental health professionals envision when they think of eating disorders. She also did not seem like a person they expected to diagnose with OCD, because stereotypes say that is not something Black people struggle with.

Counselors saw Marcia's race and shifted into race-based autopilot with their diagnoses.

Like Black men, Black women also experience stigma and marginalization, increasing their risk for a wide range of undiagnosed mental health problems, including eating disorders. Because Black women are characterized as being larger than White women on average,[10] the assumptions that they prefer being bigger and that they do not face pressure to conform to a slim body image creates the false impression that they do not develop eating disorders. Under those assumptions, when a Black woman develops an eating disorder, counselors tend toward dismissiveness, failing to recognize the disorder. As a result, Black and African American women who have an eating disorder are less likely to be accurately diagnosed and are often reluctant to seek treatment.[11]

In a study on the impact of client race on clinician detection of eating disorders, ninety-one clinicians read one of three passages about Mary, a fictional client with disturbed eating patterns.[12] Mary's ethnicity was changed in each of the passages to be Black, White, or Latinx. The clinicians were asked to assess whether Mary had a problem and to rate Mary's anxiety, depression, and eating disorder symptoms based upon what they read. The results showed that clinicians were less likely to diagnose a person of color with an eating disorder even if the symptoms were exactly the same as those presented by a White client.

The results suggest that a clinician's objectivity can be impeded by race-based stereotypes when diagnosing the presence of eating disorders. This is dangerous because a delay in diagnosis can increase the disorder's treatment resistance.

The Overdiagnosis of Disabilities in Black School-Age Boys

Tyrone was five years old when he and his mother fled from his abusive father. He and his mother moved into a public housing project where zoning rules allowed him to enroll in a predominantly White school with children from more privileged neighborhoods. Tyrone's anger at his father quickly led to anger directed at others. He was soon labeled by his teachers as a behavioral problem, and his reputation preceded him in every grade. Tyrone had problems with authority and needed to exert control over others. In fourth grade, the school psychologist diagnosed Tyrone with conduct disorder and a learning disability. He was on a trajectory toward becoming an African American boy lost in the school-to-prison pipeline, and most of his teachers were content to let that be his fate.

In fifth grade, Tyrone's teacher, who was an older White woman, took a special interest in him. She could see the nature of Tyrone's pain and anger, but she believed in him. This teacher changed Tyrone's life by motivating, affirming, and rewarding him for his efforts. Fifth grade was a year of unbelievable turnaround for Tyrone. He went on to student leadership roles. He learned that he could control his fate, and although he couldn't control other people, he could control his reactions to them. Tyrone graduated from high school on time and went on to earn bachelor, master's, and doctorate degrees. He has spent much of his life working with neighborhood children and adolescents with externalizing disorders and substance use problems.

Tyrone's behavior from kindergarten through fourth grade was misinterpreted. One person recognized and provided what Tyrone needed rather than labeling him.

When working with Black children and adolescents, counselors must find balance between underdiagnosis and overdiagnosis. Teens are frequently overlooked when it comes to depression and suicide risk, while younger children are commonly overrepresented in terms of emotional and behavioral diagnoses. Black boys bear the brunt of the uneven representation.

In 1968, Lloyd M. Dunn's seminal work brought attention to this disproportionality and recognized that special education programs may harm the self-image of these children.[13] Christopher B. Townsend's study of school counselors' perceptions and effectiveness regarding African American boys with disabilities in special education expanded on Dunn's work by examining the processes that lead to Black and African American boys being placed in special education.[14] Townsend noted that approximately fifty years after Dunn's concept was introduced, statistics from the US Department of Education's National Center for Education Statistics corroborated Dunn's claim:

> The data shows that among students ages 3 to 21 who are served by Individuals with Disabilities Education Act (IDEA) programs, Emotional Disturbance is documented as occurring at a rate of 7.4% among African American students and 7.0% among mixed-race students, while occurring at rates of only 2% to 5.5% for all other races/ethnic groups. Intellectual Disability is documented as occurring at a rate of 9.3% for African American students, while occurring at rates of only 5.2% to 6.6% for all other races.[15]

Here are some of the ways Black boys are overrepresented in clinical problems and diagnoses:[16]

- Students receiving special education are likely to identify as African American, male, urban, and from low socioeconomic backgrounds.[17]
- Black students make up about 17 percent of the nation's general student body; however, they categorically represent 33 percent of the nation's high-incidence disability categories.[18]
- Black students have greater rates of reported emotional disturbance, cognitive disorders, learning disabilities, and speech and language disorders.[19]
- The 2010 Civil Rights Data Collection reported that Black males make up 16.6 percent of special education students although they comprise only 8.5 percent of the total K–12 student population.[20]

To avoid "biasnosis," school counselors must recognize institutional biases within school systems, instrument biases in the assessments they utilize, and any personal biases affecting their interpretation of facts.

THE UNDERDIAGNOSIS OF AUTISM SPECTRUM DISORDER

B. J. was an African American single male who died by suicide at age thirty-two. To everyone who met him, he was known as friendly, kind,

loveable, witty, intelligent, self-sacrificing, and thrill-seeking. As a tod-
dler, B. J. was slow in speech development, but the nuances in his speech
were deemed to be culturally normative. Friends and teachers alike
offered normalizing statements to his parents: "It's common for African
American boys to need speech therapy. No big deal." From elementary
school onward, B. J.'s academic life was a roller-coaster ride. His parents,
both professionals, were frequently called to the school to discuss his
behavior. B. J. did not get in trouble at school for doing "bad" things, but
he had a propensity for fun, distraction, and rule-breaking oddities that
were difficult to pinpoint, and he often did not turn in his homework.

B. J.'s mom talked to his first-grade teacher about the possibility of
an attention-deficit/hyperactivity disorder (ADHD) diagnosis, but his
teacher said she was certain it was not ADHD behavior, although she
could not speculate any further about what "it" actually was. In second
grade, B. J. made honor roll one semester, but he tore up his honor roll
certificate and threw it away without taking it home. B. J.'s grades fluc-
tuated cyclically from an A-B-C report card to a C-D-F report card,
falling as soon as B. J.'s mother would try to show confidence in him and
let him do his schoolwork more independently. In school, B. J. lived in the
shadow of his sister, who was one year ahead of him and was an advanced
straight-A student in intellectually gifted and advanced placement
classes. From kindergarten through his senior year of high school, B. J.'s
teachers told his parents that his behavior was just a matter of maturity,
and he would "grow out of it" in due time.

His parents wanted so badly for him to function at an age-normative
level. B. J.'s mom suffered from undiagnosed anxiety and often became
impatient with him. She felt guilty about not being softer with him, but
her fears for his outcome fueled a vicious cycle of anxiety and knowing
that something just was not right. B. J.'s parents took him for regular
medical check-ups with one of the city's leading pediatricians, but nothing abnormal was identified. B. J.'s mom wondered if he had a learning
or developmental disability.

By middle school, it become apparent that B.J. had an exceptionally
keen sense of hearing. He was aware of certain aspects of sound that
most people weren't attuned to. At school and at church, he became

the resident audio engineer because he could set the audio equipment to deliver superior sound quality. Through middle school, high school, and beyond, he loved to be at his sound board, creating music, mixing digital sounds, and working as a D.J. His "golden ears" were like a superpower.

By the time B.J. got to high school, his mom had earned her degree in mental health counseling, working with adult populations. B.J. seemed to be doing better, so she hoped the maturity hypothesis was accurate. The possibility of ADHD came up again at the end of B.J.'s sophomore year when the school psychologist wanted to do an assessment. His mom knew, as did some of B.J.'s teachers, that B.J. would benefit from an evaluation, but his father would not consent because of the stigma and fears about Black boys being labeled.

After high school graduation, B.J. completed a few semesters at a local university and had odd jobs in restaurants here and there. He never married and he seemed to spend his adult years unable to get out of teenage behavioral patterns. By his mid-twenties, B.J. was in the throes of alcoholism, drug use, and depression. He died just shortly before receiving his first thirty-day sobriety token from his new Alcoholics Anonymous group.

After his death, his mother began to read about autism spectrum disorders, and recognized—too late—that B.J. had likely lived his whole life with undiagnosed level 1 autism. Among other things, she learned that a growing number of research studies have found that autistic youth and adults appear to have higher rates of suicidal thoughts, plans, or behaviors than non-autistic people do. As a group, their suicide risk may be two to seven times higher than the risk for youth and adults who do not have autism.[21]

B.J.'s mother will never know for sure, but she often thinks about whether her son's outcome would have been different if only she had insisted on an assessment; if teachers had not dismissed B.J.'s behavior as just an immaturity issue; if they had not defined his struggles as within normal range for Black boys; if she had addressed her own mental health and if she had recognized the impact of her generalized anxiety disorder earlier. Now she struggles with depression also, and the weight of feeling that she failed her son. The ache in her heart comes with "if" as a *constant* companion.

Evaluation Disparities for Autism Spectrum Disorder.

"Black children usually obtain a diagnosis for autism one and a half years later than White children, after many more provider visits. They are also more likely to be misdiagnosed first with intellectual disabilities and emotional and behavioral disorders, creating an even longer delay."[22] A team of researchers examining why diagnosis delays exist for Black children found that Black children were excluded from the earliest studies on children with autism. Early research focused primarily on White male children, and White males have continued to be overrepresented in scientific studies on autism. Autism can affect anyone, but it may present differently based on race or gender. As a result, autism screenings do a better job of identifying autism in White male children because that is the group represented in most studies.

One hundred and sixty Black parents and caretakers took part in a 2021 study led by Torica Exume at Florida Atlantic University that found that "Black children diagnosed with autism tend to have more severe clinical presentation than White children, suggesting that Black children with less impairing symptoms may be missed altogether. These diagnostic disparities may reflect providers' racial biases."[23] More research is needed within the Black community, especially on autism. In the meantime, counselors must pay close attention to possible biases in their case conceptualizations, diagnoses, referrals, and interventions, to prevent Black children like B. J. from being overlooked.

UNDERESTIMATING BLACK SUICIDE RISK

B. J. was one of approximately 47,000 people who died by suicide in 2019. That year, suicide was the second leading cause of death for all people between the ages of ten and thirty-four.[24] Within those total numbers, African American suicide rates were among the most alarming.

African American Suicide Risk

Interestingly, the Centers for Disease Control and Prevention (CDC) reported that the national suicide rate decreased from 14.2 per 100,000 individuals in 2018 to 13.9 per 100,000 individuals in 2019, the first year-over-year decrease since 1999.[25] Unfortunately, the overall rates of African American suicide do not follow that trend. In fact, African American suicide has been on the rise since 1965,[26] but the trend was not given much attention until recently. Between 2014 and 2019, rates of suicide among Black people in the United States increased by 30 percent, from 5.7 to 7.4 per 100,000 individuals.[27] According to the Suicide Prevention Resource Center, between 2011 and 2020, the suicide rate among Black men was three times that of Black women.[28]

According to CDC data, the prevalence of suicide attempts among Black teenagers increased 73 percent between 1991 and 2017.[29] A Congressional Black Caucus report entitled *Ring the Alarm: The Crisis of Black Youth Suicide in America* noted the increasing trend of Black adolescent suicides and called for the nation's attention:

> While research has [also] shown climbing rates for youth from other racial and ethnic groups, this trend in Black youth runs counter to historical data showing lower rates of suicide among Black Americans. It challenges the public perception that Black youth simply do not commit suicide. Additional research about suicidal behaviors has raised questions about whether the path from suicidal thoughts to attempts is well understood in Black youth, and whether we have the knowledge and tools to intervene before the worst happens.[30]

Suicidal thoughts are frequently overlooked among adolescents, particularly in African American households: "In a large-scale study, it was found that half of the caregivers were unaware that their child had thoughts about suicide, and rates of both parental unawareness and adolescent denial of suicidal thoughts were higher among racial minority families (most of whom were Black)."[31]

What's Behind the Rising African American Suicide Rate?

Dr. Patrice Harris, the first Black woman to be elected president of the American Medical Association, suggested five factors that may be contributing to the increase in suicides among Black Americans: social media pressure, mental health stigma, inaccessible treatment, racism and discrimination, and exposure to violence.[32]

Social Media Ramps Up Pressure to Fit In

Social media creates pressure to portray the image of a perfect life, and young people are especially vulnerable to this strain. This pressure can adversely affect a person's sense of self, identity, and belonging. Cyberbullying on social media was found to be a common form of harassment experienced by Black adolescents. Studies show that cyberbullying is associated with increased suicidal ideation among both Black and White people.[33]

Mental Health Stigma Impedes Black People from Seeking Help

The stigma associated with mental health in Black communities continues to be a barrier to seeking help. The main concern for Black men—being seen as weak if they seek help—still influences negative perceptions about counseling. Equally significant is the notion of the Strong Black Woman who demonstrates tireless strength and cares for others without limits or help. Each of these identity representations creates idealistic images that people want to attain. Harris calls for people to be intentional about addressing mental health stigma and reframing how mental health issues are discussed in Black communities.[34]

Treatment Is Often Less Accessible to Black People

Many Black families live in impoverished areas where financial and educational resources for mental health are slim. The limited availability of culturally conscious providers only makes matters worse.[35] For people who want and would utilize treatment services, this is a true treatment barrier.

Black People Continually Face Racism and Discrimination

Structural racism and daily discrimination, whether experienced personally or indirectly through mainstream media, have a significant role in mental health. Bias, lack of culturally appropriate training, and other forms of systemic discrimination can lead to hopelessness and take a toll on a person's mental health and overall well-being. Harris calls for the dismantling of the racist systems that cause many of these mental health issues in the first place.[36]

Violence and Accumulative Trauma

Like racism, violence yields undesirable emotional outcomes in the lives of children. Although not all Black people live in impoverished and violent communities, research suggests that they are generally exposed to disproportionately more violence than Whites.[37]

Researchers have recently highlighted the divergence between lower depression diagnoses and rising rates of suicide completion among Black boys and men. The number draws attention to the underdiagnosis of depression in this population.

The Underdiagnosis of Depression in Black Men

As discussed earlier, Black men appear to have a lower rate of depression than White men. The *DSM-5-TR* symptom criteria for major depressive disorder are as follows:[38] The individual must be continuously experiencing at least five or more of the following symptoms for at least two weeks.

1. A depressed mood most of the day, every day

2. A loss of interest in all or almost all activities

3. Weight loss or a loss of appetite

4. Insomnia (a lack of sleep) or hypersomnia (increased sleep)

5. Constant fatigue

6. Feelings of worthlessness and inappropriate self-guilt

7. Suicidal thoughts or ideations

8. A reduced ability to think, focus, or concentrate

9. Psychomotor agitation (anxious restlessness that is typically not related to any event going on)

10. Psychomotor retardation may also be present. (This is the opposite of psychomotor agitation. The individual's thoughts, movements, and cognitive function are slow.)

It was once believed that all people experienced depressive symptoms in the same way. As research has evolved, the validity and reliability of *DSM 5-TR* parameters for depression in Black men is a matter of debate. Black men experience depressive symptoms with long-lasting severity and persistence, and a modest amount of research indicates that Black men characterize depression symptoms using terminology and traits that differ from those found in the *DSM-5-TR* definition of depression.[39]

A team of researchers employed a stakeholder-driven, community-engaged process for understanding Black men's depression. The stakeholders included Black men, Black women, and primary care providers. The study identified sixty-eight characteristics of Black men's depression that were categorized into six clusters: (1) physical states, (2) emotional states, (3) diminished drive, (4) internal conflicts, (5) communication with others, and (6) social pressures. Tables 8.1 through 8.6 show the identified depression characteristics for Black men.[40]

Table 8.1: Physical States

1 High blood pressure
2 Self-harm or suicidal behavior
3 Binge eating
4 Insomnia
5 Oversleeping or sleeping frequently
6 Heart palpitations
7 Weight loss
8 Weight gain

THE PHYSICAL STATES CLUSTER DESCRIBES PHYSICAL MANIFESTATIONS OF NEGATIVE AFFECT, INCLUDING SOMATIC SYMPTOMS, CLINICAL DIAGNOSES, CLINICAL SYMPTOMS, AND WEIGHT CHANGES.

SOURCE: LESLIE B. ADAMS ET AL., "REFINING BLACK MEN'S DEPRESSION MEASUREMENT USING PARTICIPATORY APPROACHES: A CONCEPT MAPPING STUDY," *BMC PUBLIC HEALTH* 21, NO. 1 (2021).

Table 8.2: Emotional States

1	Not able to get up and go
2	Lack of motivation
3	Anger
4	Feeling sick
5	Low self-esteem
6	Being stagnant or stuck in life
7	Laziness
8	Feeling out of control
9	Feeling irritated or agitated
10	Feeling fatigued
11	Feeling hopeless
12	Feeling frustrated
13	Bursts of crying
14	Not feeling like yourself
15	Worry
16	Anxiety

THE EMOTIONAL STATES CLUSTER DESCRIBES BOTH THE INTERNALIZING AND EXTERNALIZING EMOTIONAL EXPERIENCES OF DEPRESSED MOOD.

SOURCE: LESLIE B. ADAMS ET AL., "REFINING BLACK MEN'S DEPRESSION MEASUREMENT USING PARTICIPATORY APPROACHES: A CONCEPT MAPPING STUDY," *BMC PUBLIC HEALTH* 21, NO. 1 (2021).

Table 8.3: Internal Conflict

1	Having a pessimistic outlook or negative mindset
2	Feeling guilty
3	Feeling unqualified (impostor syndrome)
4	Having a heightened sense of fear or dread
5	Not feeling supported by the Black community
6	Not feeling valued for your work or not seeing the benefits of hard work over time
7	Feeling like things are "off"
8	Feeling attacked or defensive
9	Change in mood overtime as men age
10	Feeling helpless due to the aging process (increased reliance on assistance from others)
11	Numbness, melancholy, or lack of engagement that can be observed by others (e.g. "There's no joy in your eyes.")

THE INTERNAL CONFLICT CLUSTER INCLUDES BRAINSTORMED STATEMENTS THAT NAMED INTERNALIZED SENTIMENTS AND INTERNALIZED STANDINGS IN THE BLACK COMMUNITY.

SOURCE: LESLIE B. ADAMS ET AL., "REFINING BLACK MEN'S DEPRESSION MEASUREMENT USING PARTICIPATORY APPROACHES: A CONCEPT MAPPING STUDY," *BMC PUBLIC HEALTH* 21, NO. 1 (2021).

Table 8.4: Communication with Others

---

1 Unable to communicate properly (delayed or ignored emails, calls, text, etc.)

2 Isolation from others (friends, family, romantic partners, etc.)

3 Discouraging others (misery loves company)

4 Unclear or limited communication (unclear or limited communication (short verbal responses, unclear body language, etc.)

5 Feeling hopeless due to prolonged exposure to state violence against Black people (police shootings on social media, news coverage, etc.)

6 Blunted emotional expression or flat affect (not crying, no facial changes, etc.)

7 Withdrawal from everyday activities, hobbies, interest, etc.

8 Not able to maintain romantic relationships

9 Stuffing down emotions

10 Ignoring support from others

11 Personality or mood changes in romantic relationships

12 Volatile behavior toward others

13 Sharing emotions through indirect forms of communication (writing long emotional status updates on social media, letters, emails, etc.)

14 Blaming others for issues

15 Only reflecting or reminiscing on certain life stages (adolescence, early adulthood, etc.)

16 Change in sexual behavior in relationships (loss of interest, aggression, etc.)

17 Re-establishing relationships with past acquaintances (friends, romantic partners, etc.)

18 Seeking closure with others; wrapping up loose ends

THE COMMUNICATION WITH OTHERS CLUSTER INCLUDED EIGHTEEN BRAINSTORMED STATEMENTS ABOUT THE CHALLENGES OF MAINTAINING INTERPERSONAL COMMUNICATION (VERBAL AND NON-VERBAL PATTERNS) WITH DEPRESSED MOOD.

SOURCE: LESLIE B. ADAMS ET AL., "REFINING BLACK MEN'S DEPRESSION MEASUREMENT USING PARTICIPATORY APPROACHES: A CONCEPT MAPPING STUDY," *BMC PUBLIC HEALTH* 21, NO. 1 (2021).

Table 8.5: Social Pressures

1	Not being able to keep up appearances (different clothes, shoes, etc. than peers)
2	Fear of the unknown consequences of today's political environment
3	Adherence to norms of competition with other men (feeling the need to do better than the other guy, etc.)
4	Adherence to cultural norms of success and power (keeping up with the Joneses, having a large salary, high-powered job, etc.)
5	Constant strain to do what you have to do to survive (support kids, pay bills, etc.)
6	Lack of work-life balance
7	Ignoring physical symptoms (injuries, pain, discomfort, etc.)
8	Excessive engagement in activities that improve outward appearance (overexercise, overspending, etc.)
9	Seeking happiness through accumulated materials (clothes, shoes, etc.)
10	Increased attendance at religious institutions (church, mosque, etc.)

THE SOCIAL PRESSURES CLUSTER REPRESENTS ISSUES RELATED TO THE STRAINS ASSOCIATED WITH ACHIEVING TRADITIONAL MALE GENDER ROLES.

SOURCE: LESLIE B. ADAMS ET AL., "REFINING BLACK MEN'S DEPRESSION MEASUREMENT USING PARTICIPATORY APPROACHES: A CONCEPT MAPPING STUDY," *BMC PUBLIC HEALTH* 21, NO. 1 (2021).

Table 8.6: Diminished Drive

1	Untidy or messy appearance (home, personal hygiene, etc.)
2	Not able to complete tasks
3	Not able to provide for family
4	Not able to complete life goals (finishing school, getting a job, traveling, etc)
5	Excessive substance use (marijuana, cigarettes, alcohol)

THE DIMINISHED DRIVE CLUSTER INCLUDES FIVE BRAINSTORMED STATEMENTS RELATED TO UNFINISHED BUSINESS AND UNTAPPED POTENTIAL OF BLACK MEN.

SOURCE: LESLIE B. ADAMS ET AL., "REFINING BLACK MEN'S DEPRESSION MEASUREMENT USING PARTICIPATORY APPROACHES: A CONCEPT MAPPING STUDY," *BMC PUBLIC HEALTH* 21, NO. 1 (2021).

Do commonly used assessments capture these depression characteristics?
This study compared the six clusters in the participant results against three current assessments for depression: Beck's Depression Inventory (BDI), Center for Epidemiological Studies Depression (CESD) scale, and the Patient Health Questionnaire-9 (PHQ-9). Although each of these instruments includes portions of the participants' lists, none of the three captures all six of the depression clusters identified in the research study.[41]

Counselors must be cognizant of the evidence that Black men's depression experiences may be articulated differently. The commonly used depression assessments may not be capturing the actual prevalence of depression in Black men. Because of the differences expressed in subtle cultural nuances and wording, Black male depression may be grossly underreported. If counselors can ask clarifying questions using the type of culturally viable language in the study results, they will gain a more accurate clinical case conceptualization and diagnosis.

The researchers noted that primary care physicians may be the most accessible and first point of contact for many Black men with depression symptoms.[42] Medically unclear somatization may indicate that a client needs further screening or assessment. All providers, including those in medicine and behavioral health, must remember that Black men's depressive symptoms may be expressed in ways that are different from the *DSM-5-TR* language due to cultural and masculine perceptions of strength and weakness. Lastly, counselors, pastors, and other concerned individuals in the community should pay special attention to how Black men articulate aspects of their everyday lives and their social strain.

Depression in Young Black Men
Other research focusing specifically on *young* Black men identified other challenges to using traditional clinical definitions of depression with this population.[43] Restrictive emotionality is common among young Black men because expression of painful emotions is deemed to be feminine. Young Black men also dismiss feelings of depression by accepting that hardship is "just a fact of life." Consistent with the aforementioned study, traditional conceptualizations are not aligned with their understanding

of depression. The stigmatization of mental health is likewise a prevalent factor for Black men because of the embarrassment, shame, and secrecy it brings.

Breaking the Cycle

The general patterns of diagnostic bias identified in the literature are worrisome, to say the least. Counselors must raise the bar and address "biasnosis" as an ethical concern and a matter of racial justice in mental health. Only then will our profession move toward viable, culturally astute care for *all* people.

NOTES

1. Lucius M. Lampton, "Samuel Adolphus Cartwright," Mississippi Encyclopedia (April 13, 2018), https://mississippiencyclopedia.org/entries/samuel-adolphus-cartwright; Samuel Cartwright, "Diseases and Peculiarities of the Negro Race," *De Bow's Review* XI (1851), https://www.pbs.org/wgbh/aia/part4/4h3106t.html; Oxford Reference Online, s.v. "dysaesthesia aethiopis (*n*)," accessed April 18, 2023, https://www.oxfordreference.com/view/10.1093/oi/authority.20110803095737938; *Oxford Reference Online*, s.v. "drapetomania (*n*)," accessed April 18, 2023, https://www.oxfordreference.com/view/10.1093/oi/authority.20110803095730308.

2. Cartwright, "Diseases"; Oxford Reference, "dysaesthesia."

3. Lampton, "Samuel"; Cartwright, "Diseases"; *Oxford,* "dysaesthesia"; *Oxford,* "drapetomania."

4. Cartwright, "Diseases."

5. "Racism and Mental Health," Mental Health America, accessed April 10, 2023, https://mhanational.org/racism-and-mental-health.

6. "Schizophrenia," National Institute of Mental Health (U.S. Department of Health and Human Services), accessed April 12, 2023, https://www.nimh.nih.gov/health/statistics/schizophrenia#:~:text=Schizophrenia-,Definition,be%20both%20severe%20and%20disabling.

7. *Diagnostic and Statistical Manual of Mental Disorders,* 5th ed. (Washington, DC: American Psychiatric Association Publishing, 2022).

8. "Racism and Mental Health."

9. "Racism and Mental Health."

10. Peter T. Katzmarzyk et al., "Ethnic-Specific BMI and Waist Circumference Thresholds," *Obesity* 19, no. 6 (June 2011): 1272–78, https://doi.org/10.1038/oby.2010.319.

11. Lauren Muhlheim, "The Impact of Race and Racism on Eating Disorders," Verywell Mind, May 9, 2022, https://www.verywellmind.com/race-racism-and-eating-disorders-5076344.

12. Kathryn H. Gordon et al., "The Impact of Client Race on Clinician Detection of Eating Disorders," *Behavior Therapy* 37, no. 4 (2006): 319–25, https://doi.org/10.1016/j.beth.2005.12.002.

13. Lloyd M. Dunn, "Special Education for the Mildly Retarded—Is Much of It Justifiable?," *Exceptional Children* 35, no. 1 (1968): 5–22, https://doi.org/10.1177/001440296803500101.

14. Christopher B. Townsend, "A Grounded Theory Study of School Counselors' Perceptions and Effectiveness Regarding African American Boys with Disabilities Who Are Disproportionately Represented in Special Education" (PhD. diss., North Carolina Agricultural and Technical State University, 2018).

15. "Digest of Education Statistics, 2016," National Center for Education Statistics (NCES) Home Page, a Part of the U.S. Department of Education, accessed April 12, 2023, https://nces.ed.gov/programs/digest/d16/tables/dt16_204.50.asp; Kristen Faye Linton, "Differential Ratings of Specific Behaviors of African Americans Children in Special Education," *Child and Adolescent Social Work Journal* 32, no. 3 (December 2014): 229–35, https://doi.org/10.1007/s10560-014-0363-3.

16. LaVerne Hanes Collins and Alfonso L. Ferguson, "Culturally Responsive Counseling for Clients of African American, African, and Afro-Caribbean Descent," in *Multicultural Counseling: Responding with Cultural Humility, Empathy, and Advocacy,* ed. LaTonya M. Summers and Lotes Nelson (New York, NY: Springer Publishing, 2023), 61.

17. Townsend, "A Grounded Theory Study"; Alfredo J. Artiles et al., "Justifying and Explaining Disproportionality, 1968–2008: A Critique of Underlying Views of Culture," *Exceptional Children* 76, no. 3 (2010): 279–99, https://doi.org/10.1177/001440291007600303; Martha J. Coutinho et al., "Gender and Sociodemographic Factors and the Disproportionate Identification of Culturally and Linguistically Diverse Students with Emotional Disturbance," *Behavioral Disorders* 27, no. 2 (2002): 109–25, https://doi.org/10.1177/019874290202700202.

18. Townsend, "A Grounded Theory Study"; Gwendolyn Cartledge and Charles Dukes, "Disproportionality of African American Children in Special Education: Definition and Dimensions," in *The Sage Handbook of African American Education,* ed. Linda C. Tillman (Thousand Oaks, CA: Sage Publications, 2008).

19. Townsend, "A Grounded Theory Study."

20. Townsend, "A Grounded Theory Study."

21. T. Hirvikoski et al., "Individual Risk and Familial Liability for Suicide Attempt and Suicide in Autism: A Population-Based Study," Psychological Medicine 50, no. 9 (2019): 1463–74, doi: 10.1017/S0033291719001405; Lisa A. Croen et al., "The Health Status of Adults on the Autism Spectrum," Autism 19, no. 7 (2015): 814–23, https://doi.org/10.1177/1362361315577517; Mu-Hong Chen et al., "Risk of Suicide Attempts among Adolescents and Young Adults with Autism Spectrum Disorder," Journal of Clinical Psychiatry 78, no. 9 (2017), doi: 10.4088/JCP.16m11100; Anne V. Kirby et al., "A 20-Year Study of Suicide Death in a Statewide Autism Population," *Autism Research* 12, no. 4 (2019): 658–66, https://doi.org/10.1002/aur.2076; L. O'Halloran, P. Coey, and C. Wilson, "Suicidality in Autistic Youth: A Systematic Review and Meta-Analysis," *Clinical Psychology Review* 93 (2022): 102144, https://doi.org/10.1016/j.cpr.2022.102144.

22. Katie Hyson, "New Research Suggests Delays in Autism Diagnosis for Black Children May Reflect Providers' Racial Biases Report for America," *WUFT News*, February 23, 2022, https://www.wuft.org/news/2022/02/18/autism/#:~:text=Black%20children%20usually%20obtain%20a,creating%20an%20even%20longer%20delay.

23. Hyson, "New Research."

24. Marina Sarris, "Autism and the Troubling Risk of Suicide," *SPARK for Autism*, September 7, 2022, https://sparkforautism.org/discover_article/autism-suicide-risk.

25. Rajeev Ramchand, Joshua A. Gordon, and Jane L. Pearson, "Trends in Suicide Rates by Race and Ethnicity in the United States," *JAMA Network Open* 4, no. 5 (May 26, 2021), doi:10.1001/jamanetworkopen.2021.11563.

26. Sean Joe and Mark S. Kaplan, "Suicide among African American Men," *Suicide and Life-Threatening Behavior* 31 (January 26, 2001): 106–21, https://doi.org/10.1521/suli.31.1.5.106.24223; Marisa Spann et al., "Suicide and African American Teenagers: Risk Factors and Coping Mechanisms," *Suicide and Life-Threatening Behavior* 36, no. 5 (October 2006): 553–68, https://doi.org/10.1521/suli.2006.36.5.553.

27. Ramchand et al., "Trends in Suicide Rates."

28. Maia Niguel Hoskin, "5 Reasons Suicide Is on the Rise in Black Communities," *EverydayHealth.com,* May 2022, https://www.everydayhealth.com/emotional-health/reasons-suicide-is-on-the-rise-in-the-black-community-according-to-a-psychiatrist.

29. Michael A. Lindsey et al., "Trends of Suicidal Behaviors among High School Students in the United States: 1991–2017," *Pediatrics* 144, no. 5 (November 2019), https://doi.org/10.1542/peds.2019-1187.

30. Bonnie Watson Coleman, *Ring the Alarm: The Crisis of Black Youth Suicide in America: A Report to Congress from the Congressional Black Caucus*, 2019, https://watsoncoleman.house.gov/imo/media/doc/full_taskforce_report.pdf.

31. Lindsey et al., "Trends of Suicidal Behaviors among High School Students," 19.

32. Hoskin, "5 Reasons."

33. Hoskin, "5 Reasons."

34. Hoskin, "5 Reasons."

35. Hoskin, "5 Reasons."

36. Hoskin, "5 Reasons."

37. Hoskin, "5 Reasons."

38. *Diagnostic and Statistical Manual.*

39. Leslie B. Adams et al., "Refining Black Men's Depression Measurement Using Participatory Approaches: A Concept Mapping Study," *BMC Public Health* 21, no. 1 (2021), https://doi.org/10.1186/s12889-021-11137-5. This is the source document for this entire section.

40. Adams et al., "Refining Black Men's Depression Measurement."

41. Adams et al., "Refining Black Men's Depression Measurement."

42. Adams et al., "Refining Black Men's Depression Measurement."

43. Danielle E. K. Perkins, "Challenges to Traditional Clinical Definitions of Depression in Young Black Men," *American Journal of Men's Health* 8, no. 1 (August 2013): 74–81, https://doi.org/10.1177/1557988313494234.

PART IV
OVERLOOKED LOSSES

CHAPTER 9

The Impact of a Shorter Life Expectancy for Black Americans

The idea is to die young, as late as possible.

—Ashley Montagu

In the United States, there is a long-standing and well-documented disparity between the life expectancy of Black people and that of White people.[1] Much of that disparity could be reduced and many preventable early deaths could be avoided if it were not for the existence of vast racial and socioeconomic inequities. Black people die younger because of the complex interactions of many factors, including poverty and structural racism—known culprits of poor health and mortality.

Life expectancy reflects the average number of years a newborn would be expected to live, based on current mortality rates. Life expectancy, age-adjusted death rates, and infant mortality form a trilogy of indicators about the overall health and well-being of any population. These measures provide summary information that shows the United States ranking lower than comparable peer nations in health outcomes. In general, longevity is extended in the presence of better living conditions and access to health care–related resources throughout the life span.[2]

The burden of racism has been shown to decrease a person's life span by activating inflammatory and disease-causing genes.[3] Research shows that "differential exposure to racial discrimination may contribute to racial disparities in health outcomes in part by activating threat-related molecular programs that stimulate inflammation and contribute to increased risk of chronic illnesses."[4]

Whether directly or indirectly, racism leads to greater poverty, unhealthy living environments, and less access to quality health care. Those conditions lead to fewer physician visits, ill health, poorer pregnancy care, nutritional disparities, and ultimately a shorter life expectancy.[5] Recognizing the impact of racism and concluding that their loved one may have lived longer in a world without health inequities and racial disparities adds a layer of complexity to the emotional weight of the grieving family.[6]

LIFE IS SHORTER WHEN YOU'RE BLACK

Black people have the highest mortality and lowest survival rates of any racial or ethnic group for most forms of cancer.[7] They also have higher mortality rates for other leading causes of death, including heart disease, stroke, and diabetes. Non-Hispanic Black women are 3.55 times more likely to die during pregnancy and the first six weeks postpartum compared to non-Hispanic White women.[8] These disease and mortality rates make early loss a common experience in Black communities.

> Standard views of grief do not address how African Americans are impacted by the substantial difference in life expectancy between Blacks and Whites.

In 2020, the average life expectancy at birth for all race and ethnicity groups in the United States was 77.0 years. However, non-Hispanic Black life expectancy was only 71.5 years, representing a 5.5-year disadvantage compared to the overall population, and a negative differential of almost 6 years compared to non-Hispanic Whites. The non-Hispanic Asian population had the highest life expectancy at birth (83.6 years), followed by the Hispanic (77.9) and non-Hispanic White (77.4) populations. The shortest life expectancy (67.1) was found among the non-Hispanic

American Indian/Alaska Native population.[9] For men, the disparity is even more pronounced: Seven years separate the life expectancies of non-Hispanic African American men (67.8 years) and non-Hispanic White men (74.8 years).[10]

THE RISK OF EARLY DEATH EXPOSURE

According to a study conducted by the Population Research Center at the University of Texas at Austin, the death of family members is an overlooked source of racial disadvantage in the United States that is damaging to the long-term mental and physical health of Black Americans. Numerous life cycle outcomes are adversely affected by these losses due to the debilitating impact of grief and other related factors that carry risks across the entire life span.[11]

The study revealed that Blacks experience more family member deaths at an early age than Whites. By the age of thirty, a Black person was twice as likely to have already faced the loss of two or more family members. By age sixty-five, they were 90 percent more likely to have already experienced four or more family deaths. Compare that to Whites, who by age sixty-five were 50 percent more likely to have *never* experienced a family member death.

Overall, Blacks had a higher probability of losing a mother from early childhood through young adulthood, a father in their mid-teen years, and a sibling in their teen years. Blacks also had a higher probability of losing a child before the age of thirty. Things begin to level out by age seventy, when Whites and Blacks have more equitable experiences of loss.

This study assessed loss by age cohort group. Looking at the cumulative risk of specific family member deaths for Black and White respondents, the differences are notable in both younger and older cohorts, and the disparities begin early in life.

For people born between 1980 and 1984, the study found that by age ten, Blacks were 20 percent more likely to have lost a sibling, more than twice as likely to have lost their father, and three times more likely to have lost their mother. By age twenty, a Black person was a little more than twice as likely to have lost a child, and by age thirty, that likelihood grew to 2.5 times the average.[12]

Looking at people in older cohorts born from 1900 to 1965, the study found that by age twenty a Black person was twice as likely to have lost their mother and had about a 50 percent greater risk of losing their father, compared to a White person of the same age. Between age fifty and sixty, a Black person was two times more likely to lose a child, and between age fifty and seventy, a Black person was over three times more likely to lose a child. By age sixty, a Black person was 50 percent more likely to lose a sibling and nearly twice as likely to have lost a spouse, again compared to a White person of the same age.[13]

The study considered the impact of repeated bereavements and focused on racial differences in life course exposure to the death of family members, which may be central to processes of cumulative disadvantage associated with race. Bereavement is a risk factor for diverse and inter-woven life outcomes. With Black Americans more likely than Whites to experience the loss of multiple family members beginning in childhood and continuing through midlife and beyond, the risk factors are present early in life. The pain and grief of losing immediate family, extended family, friends, and other significant people can be exacerbated by the widespread mass media and social media coverage of the deaths of other Black Americans. The news reports of Black people dying as a result of police brutality and gang-related violence almost certainly contribute to collective loss and feelings of personal vulnerability, even if their own loved one died of natural causes.

Early Parental Loss

A greater share of young African Americans will not have reached adult-hood when they lose a parent. Childhood parental loss has been linked to depression in adulthood and behavioral and emotional issues in teens.[14] Children find themselves displaced from the familiarity of home as they move in with another relative. That caregiver—often a grandparent or aunt/uncle—is also facing their own significant loss, which places limits on their emotional availability for the child. Additional stressors include financial insecurity and reluctance to form another strong attachment bond for fear of experiencing more loss.

Regardless of the cause and circumstances, the death of a parent and the resulting adversities after that loss can profoundly disrupt a child's life, adversely affect their health, alter their developmental trajectory, and lead to a higher mortality risk when compared to non-bereaved children.[15] Programs and supports that encourage adaptive resilience can help minimize the long-term adverse consequences, but bereaved youth are often overlooked and under-resourced, even without considering the additional disadvantages encountered by many Black children.[16]

A parent's death often requires that older children take responsibility for their younger siblings and household tasks that would otherwise be handled by the parent. The early loss of a parent also means that a child will miss that parent's role modeling through the various stages of life, such as menopause and retirement.[17] Children may feel angry and be misunderstood and labeled as a behavioral problem as they grieve. Any disruption they cause may be a reflection of the relational and emotional upheaval for which they do not have the vocabulary or capacity to verbalize.

For Black midlife adults who have lost a parent before the age of seventeen, research shows more relationship strain with their own adult children, an issue not found for non-Hispanic White midlife adults. This suggests that the development of policies, programs, and interventions to support bereaved children may bring benefits later in life for their relationships with their own children. In midlife, counseling that addresses physical and emotional problems from a loss perspective may be viable for adults who experienced the death of a parent in their early years.[18]

Loss of a Child

The death of a child of any race or ethnicity—and at any age—is a family and community tragedy. Whether from stillbirth, infant death, illness, accident, suicide, or murder, the experience of child loss is an unusually difficult and agonizing challenge, and the reorientation process is daunting. Once again, statistics for Black American children are disproportionate.

African American children are more likely to die at birth or soon thereafter.[19] In 2020 and 2021, non-Hispanic Black children had higher death rates from COVID-19 (0.4 and 1.2) than Hispanic (0.3 and 0.6) and non-Hispanic White (0.1 and 0.4) children.[20]

Black children do not fare well with accidents either. According to The Centers for Disease Control and Prevention, despite overall decreases in child unintentional injury death rates from 2010 to 2019, rates increased among some groups, including Black children. Motor vehicle death rates among Black children increased by 9 percent while rates among White children decreased by 24 percent. Poisoning death rates increased by 37 percent among Black children while rates among White children decreased by 24 percent. Drowning death rates were 2.6 times higher among Black children aged five to nine years and 3.6 times higher among Black children aged ten to fourteen years, when compared with White children of the same age.[21]

The American Academy of Child and Adolescent Psychiatry reports that suicide among Black youth has risen faster than for any other racial or ethnic group in the past two decades. For Black males ten to nineteen years old, suicide rates have increased by 60 percent.[22] Younger Black children between five and twelve years old are twice as likely to die by suicide compared to their White peers.[23]

Homicide is a leading cause of death for children in the United States, with the overall rate increasing an average of 4.3 percent every year for the last decade. Black boys died from homicide more frequently than any other group.[24]

Parents may tend to lack trust in the health care system after losing a child and thus may avoid seeking professional help for their own grief and loss or refuse needed treatment services. Researchers have found that bereaved parents struggle to find a balance between wanting to express their emotions and worrying about disclosing those feelings in the presence of someone they consider to be critical. Grieving parents frequently believe that others would be uncomfortable with conversations about their loss, so they rely on emotional support from people who share a similar experience.[25]

Early Loss of a Spouse

Because they have a shorter life expectancy than a White person, a Black married person at any age is more likely to become widowed. Navigating the death of a spouse at a young age is exceptionally challenging. Driven by the desire to grow old together, couples come together with dreams of raising children and taking grandchildren to the park together. Society expects people to lose a spouse late in life. So people often do not know what to say or do when a young spouse dies, creating tension and awkwardness in the most well-intentioned expressions of compassion.

The early loss of a spouse leaves a person feeling cheated. Life did not give their partnership the same longevity that others have enjoyed. Other widows and widowers are older and in a different stage of life. Whether the cause of death was sudden and unexpected or followed a period of illness, the loss does not come with a large same-age peer group to normalize the experience. Older widows and widowers are likely to have peer group similarity with spousal loss, but young bereaved spouses tend to feel more isolated in their experience. Meanwhile, the expectation is that they (and their children) will move on and "find someone new." If the bereaved spouse eventually finds a new partner, remarriage following bereavement can often produce an awkward three-way dynamic. The remarried person may choose to have some level of continuing bond with the deceased spouse while still desiring to form a relationship in which their new spouse feels secure.

However, finding someone new is not usually paramount. Immediate tasks include supporting the children through their grief, reorganizing finances, managing identity change, determining if relocation is necessary, preparing to raise the children alone, managing exhaustion and sadness, navigating the expectations of the deceased spouse's parents or siblings, and managing any stigma that may accompany a taboo cause of death like suicide or a communicable disease. What a young, bereaved spouse needs most is the freedom to talk about their pain without any expectation of a quick recovery.

Early Loss of a Sibling

To understand how the loss of a sibling might affect a person, it is important to first understand what makes the sibling experience unique. It is also important to identify the specifics that set the loss of a sibling apart from the loss of a parent or other loved one.[26] A sibling loss is a loss of an equal, a peer in the family, even if there is a wide age gap between siblings. When working with an African American child who is grieving the loss of a sibling, counselors should explore the child's relationship with the deceased. What kind of relationship did the surviving person have with the deceased sibling? What is their birth order and the age span between them? How many other siblings are in the family? Does the bereaved child feel any sense of guilt or responsibility for the death? What things will change now for the surviving child? Did/will the child attend the funeral or memorial for their sibling? Is this the child's first close family loss? If not, who else has died before and what kind of relationship did the child have with the earlier deceased person? How did the child cope with that previous loss?

These are questions that put the child's loss into context and give attention to the child's grief. When one sibling dies at a young age, the remaining siblings are sometimes overlooked in the mourning process as attention goes to the parents, especially the mother. This minimizes the significance of sibling loss and leads some children to hide their pain from their parents in an effort to protect the parents from further sadness.[27] Culturally sensitive counselors will look at all of these family dynamics through a cultural lens in order to help the child.

Loss of Extended Family and "Like Family"

African American family life is centered on kinship relationships and a collectivistic approach to community. This kinship had its roots in Africa and continued to be a survival norm in slavery as families were split apart on both African and American soil. A culture of non-biological family ties developed, creating "just-like-family" relationships among people unrelated by birth or marriage. However, the tie of a "just-like-family" relationship holds the same value as that of nuclear and biological family. Such relationships might be described as being of secondary importance in White communities, where a client's loss would be minimized or dismissed because the deceased person "wasn't really family" or was "only a distant cousin."[28]

The relationships between extended family members can be just as central as the relationships between close nuclear or biological family members in African American communities. The loss of one member in such a close-knit system may profoundly affect other members even when there are no blood ties,[29] leaving them with a grief that is disenfranchised because the broader society does not see their loss as significant enough to warrant space to grieve or other resources such as bereavement leave from work. Thus, their grief may be especially prolonged or complicated.

Grief Work in Counseling

Standard views of grief do not address how African Americans are impacted by the substantial difference in life expectancy between Blacks and Whites in the United States. For Black Americans, shorter life spans and higher mortality rates create an overlooked source of racial disadvantage that is damaging to long-term mental and physical health. Moreover, Black Americans are more likely to have *repeated* bereavement events that have cumulative consequences for an individual's development and sense of well-being.[30] Black Americans are also more likely to experience traumatic bereavement, wherein the loss, grief, and mourning are complicated or overpowered by the traumatic stress of the circumstances surrounding the loss.

Throughout the family life span, early death forces non-normative adjustments. Death enters the Black experience at a younger age, affecting every stage of life. A son mourns on his high school graduation day because his mother is not there to celebrate. A bride is escorted down the aisle by another family member because her father died long before her wedding day. The empty nest gets unexpectedly refilled by grandchildren, nieces, or nephews who have lost their parents. Earlier and more frequent exposure to mortality is a unique stressor that contributes to racial differences in total stress exposure and is likely to result in lifelong cumulative disadvantages for every member of a family, from the youngest to the oldest.

Counselors, do not overlook the big picture. Culturally relevant counselors demonstrate commitment to learning clinical responses and advocating for policies that address the escalating harm of racial differences and the grief and loss experienced in Black communities.[31] Black bereavement should always be viewed in terms of a series of transactional processes that are influenced by previous losses. Each loss is a part of a multigenerational family life cycle that includes the influence of the deceased and the experience of the bereaved. This facilitates Black grief work through the lens of a family systems orientation, rather than an individual orientation. But we cannot stop there: Use an ecological framework to recognize the environmental influences of discrimination, economic disadvantage, medical racism, inequitable systems, and other barriers that contribute to poor health and mortality. In so doing, we stand a chance at stemming the tide of shorter life spans for Black Americans.

NOTES

1. Nancy Breen et al., "The Effects of Residential Segregation on Black and White Mortality in the United States," *The Review of Black Political Economy* (April 2022) https://doi.org/10.1177/00346446221085487.

2. James N. Weinstein et al., *Communities in Action: Pathways to Health Equity* (Washington, DC: The National Academies Press, 2017).

3. April D. Thames et al., "Experienced Discrimination and Racial Differences in Leukocyte Gene Expression," *Psychoneuroendocrinology* 106 (2019): 277–83, https://doi.org/10.1016/j.psyneuen.2019.04.016.

4. Thames, "Experienced Discrimination," 277.

5. Paul C. Rosenblatt and Beverly R. Wallace, *African American Grief* (New York: Routledge, 2025), 1.

6. Rosenblatt and Wallace, *African American Grief*, 6.

7. Angela N. Giaquinto et al., "Cancer Statistics for African American/Black People 2022," *CA: A Cancer Journal for Clinicians* 72, no. 3 (May/June 2022): 202–29, https://doi.org/10.3322/caac.21718.

8. Marian F. MacDorman et al., "Racial and Ethnic Disparities in Maternal Mortality in the United States Using Enhanced Vital Records, 2016-2017," *American Journal of Public Health* 111, no. 9 (September 22, 2021): 1673–81, https://doi.org/10.2105/AJPH.2021.306375.

9. Elizabeth Arias and Jiaquan Q. Xu, *United States Life Tables, 2020*, 1st ed., vol. 71 (Hyattsville, MD: National Center for Health Statistics, 2022). https://dx.doi.org/10.15620/cdc:118055.

10. Arias and Xu, *United States Life Tables*, 6.

11. Debra Umberson et al., "Death of Family Members as an Overlooked Source of Racial Disadvantage in the United States," *Proceedings of the National Academy of Sciences* 114, no. 5 (2017): 915–20, https://doi.org/10.1073/pnas.1605599114.

12. Umberson, "Death of Family Members," 916.

13. Umberson, "Death of Family Members," 916.

14. Steven Pham et al., "The Burden of Bereavement: Early-Onset Depression and Impairment in Youths Bereaved by Sudden Parental Death in a 7-Year Prospective Study," *American Journal of Psychiatry* 175, no. 9 (2018): 887–96, https://doi.org/10.1176/appi.ajp.2018.17070792.

15. Michaeleen Burns et al., "Childhood Bereavement: Understanding Prevalence and Related Adversity in the United States," *American Journal of Orthopsychiatry* 90, no. 4 (January 2020): 391–405, https://doi.org/10.1037/ort0000442.

16. Burns et al., "Childhood Bereavement," 13.

17. Rosenblatt and Wallace, *African American Grief*, 2.

18. Yijung K Kim et al., "Racial Differences in Early Parental Death, Midlife Life Problems, and Relationship Strain with Adult Children," *The Journals of Gerontology: Series B* 76, no. 8 (September 13, 2021): 1617–28, https://doi.org/10.1093/geronb/gbaa232.

19. Rosenblatt and Wallace, *African American Grief*, 5.

20. "Child and Adolescent Mortality," ChildStats: Forum on Child and Family Statistics, 2022, https://www.childstats.gov/americaschildren/mortality.asp.

21. Centers for Disease Control and Prevention, "Injuries among Children and Teens," September 22, 2021, https://www.cdc.gov/injury/features/child-injury/index.html.

22. Academy of Child & Adolescent Psychiatry, "AACAP Policy Statement on Increased Suicide Among Black Youth in the U.S." https://www.aacap.org/aacap/Policy_Statements/2022/AACAP_Policy_Statement_Increased_Suicide_Among_Black_Youth_US.aspx.

23. Melinda Wenner Moyer, "Suicide Rates Rise in a Generation of Black Youth," *Scientific American*, September 29, 2021, https://www.scientificamerican.com/article/suicide-rates-rise-in-a-generation-of-black-youth.

24. Rebecca F. Wilson et al., "Trends in Homicide Rates for US Children Aged 0 to 17 Years, 1999 to 2020," *JAMA Pediatrics* 177, no. 2 (January 2023): 187, https://doi.org/10.1001/jamapediatrics.2022.4940.

25. Kimberly L. Schoonover, Larry Prokop, and Maria I. Lapid, "Valuable Informal Bereavement Support Strategies for Bereaved Parents of Stillborn, Young Children, and Adult Children: A Scoping Review," *Journal of Palliative Care* 37, no. 3 (2022): 381–400, https://doi.org/10.1177/08258597211062762.

26. Margaret M. Mahon and Mae L. Page, "Childhood Bereavement after the Death of a Sibling," *Holistic Nursing Practice* 9, no. 3 (1995): 15–26, https://doi.org/10.1097/00004650-199504000-00006.

27. Mahon and Page, "Childhood Bereavement," 20.

28. Anna Laurie and Robert A. Neimeyer, "African Americans in Bereavement: Grief as a Function of Ethnicity," *OMEGA—Journal of Death and Dying* 57, no. 2 (2008): 173–93, https://doi.org/10.2190/OM.57.2.d.

29. P. Hines, "Death and African American Culture," in *Living beyond Loss: Death in the Family*, ed. Monica McGoldrick and Froma Walsh (New York: W.W. Norton, 1991).

30. Frank J. Infurna and Axel Mayer, "Repeated Bereavement Takes Its Toll on Subjective Well-Being," *Innovation in Aging* 3, no. 4 (August 2019), https://doi.org/10.1093/geroni/igz047.

31. Umberson, "Death of Family Members," 918.

CHAPTER 10

Disenfranchised Grief and Loss

The Hidden Sorrow of Racism

Grief is a direct result of racism and intersectional violence and it affects us physically, emotionally, financially, spiritually, transnationally and transgenerationally. More importantly, not being able to fully engage in our grief is a direct outcome of chronic experiences of racist violence.

—Roberta K. Timothy

In the cycle of human development, loss is an inevitable fact of life. Counselors commonly work with grieving people and the effects of loss. Those losses come in the form of relational losses such as a death, a breakup, or an estrangement; material losses such as the loss of a home or valued possessions; immaterial losses such as one's dreams for the future; or losses of ability brought about by a decline in mental faculties or physical mobility. In all these situations, counselors invite their clients to process their feelings, accept the loss, and reimagine the future in the context of that loss.

Losses begin at an early age in both small and large ways. A child loses a tooth or a favorite toy. A family pet must be euthanized. A family moves to a new home, and the child loses their neighborhood best friend. A grandparent passes away. To ease the pain of a young child's loss, we put money under the pillow in exchange for the tooth, get a new pet, set up playdates with children in the new neighborhood, or assure them that Grandma or Grandpa is watching over them from heaven.

Grief That Goes Unnoticed

Some types of loss are overlooked: known only by those whose daily experiences include racialization and racism. Society does not allow grieving space for the losses or ensuing pain of discrimination, loss of safety, medical racism, mass incarceration, redlining, food deserts, and shorter life spans. Those are simply not losses that the general population considers.

> How does one grieve the moments of dignity loss that racism brings? How does one mourn the health effects of medical racism? How does one process the loss of opportunities that society never granted to them? How does one grieve the effects of being treated like a threat? How does one grieve over the shorter life expectancies brought about by health disparities? How does one grieve the freedom lost by the burden of suspicion that is on your race? How does one grieve the losses that are born out of ethnic bias, criminalization, stereotypes, microaggressions, broken treaties, stolen land, separation of families, devalued traditions, and tokenism?[1]

For BIPOC Americans, these are examples of ambiguous losses. Each loss cuts to the core of the human spirit and allows no room for heartache. No bereavement time from work. No one sending gift cards. No one donating meals. No one sending flowers. No rituals for mourning. No apologies for the loss. No societal acknowledgment of the tangible or intangible consequences. The very reality of a loss may be challenged: Did a loss really occur? The answer is "yes," and the result is disenfranchised grief.

Not Free to Grieve

Kenneth Doka coined the term "disenfranchised grief" to describe grief that is not publicly acknowledged by society or cannot be mourned publicly.[2] To understand disenfranchised grief, we need to understand the origin of the word. *Enfranchir* is an Old French word meaning "to make free"; disenfranchised, therefore, means "made unfree."[3]

In the study of grief and bereavement, enfranchisement applies to people who have encountered loss and have the right to experience and express feelings concerning their loss. They also can expect society to acknowledge and offer support to them. They have the freedom to publicly represent themselves as people who have suffered a loss. They may grieve publicly, mourn with others, and receive support from others. When a person's grief and bereavement are disenfranchised, however, they are denied the legitimacy and freedom of expression for their grief. The mourner's inner anguish remains concealed from public view because society does not acknowledge their need, right, or privilege to grieve openly.[4]

Generally speaking, counselors associate disenfranchised grief with losses such as the death of an abuser, infertility, post-abortion grief, the end of an illicit relationship, or separation from an incarcerated loved one. Yet counselors are not typically trained to consider disenfranchised grief related to racism and discrimination.

All grief warrants empathy, compassion, and strong social support. Unfortunately, disenfranchised grief is attached to a loss that society does not validate. As a result, the healing process may be prolonged, more difficult, or even permanently elusive. These losses are commonly nonfinite, as they may be ongoing and continuous.[5]

Grieving the Losses of Internalized Racism

Black/African American clients may also need to address the disenfranchised grief that results from internalized racism. This self-defeating form of racism involves bias against oneself or one's own ethnoracial group and typically stems from accepting negative cultural judgments that produce negative attitudes, self-degrading beliefs, or self-defeating behaviors.

Clients might need to process losses that stem from feeling less valuable than members of other groups. If at any point in their lives they have despised or undervalued the physical characteristics that are a part of their heritage, they may need to grieve that loss of self-respect.

They may also have to recover from shame-based thinking and damaged self-esteem.

CLINICAL INTERPRETATIONS

Disenfranchised grief is not a diagnosis included in the *Diagnostic and Statistical Manual of Mental Disorders*, 5th edition Text Revision (*DSM-5-TR*). It is not a symptom description, but it may account for symptoms associated with major depressive disorder; prolonged grief disorder; disorders of extreme stress not otherwise specified; adjustment disorder; post-traumatic stress disorder (PTSD); or persistent complex bereavement disorder (formerly called complicated grief disorder). Rather than place depression at the center of the treatment plan, counselors should focus on the source of grief and see if the client is interested in working through any disenfranchised grief and processing the loss from that perspective.

This method recognizes the unique problem created by disenfranchised grief: "*Unlike* other grief, the experience of disenfranchised race-based grief is typically not even recognized as such by those who live with it. *Like* other grief, it is characterized by feelings of anger, anxiety, and depression. Often those symptoms become the diagnosis of record because the disenfranchised grief of racism gets overlooked."[6]

If a Black/African American client suffers from unrecognized disenfranchised grief, the counselor may miss the mark if their clinical interventions are aimed at the wrong target (e.g., generalized anxiety disorder) without addressing the underlying disenfranchised grief. An even greater disservice to the client occurs if the counselor avoids discussing the grief of racism and further disenfranchises the pain of the client's losses.

Disenfranchised grief leaves a person feeling unnoticed in their pain, which can intensify feelings of anger and invalidation. Charles Corr describes the bias and marginalization inherent in disenfranchised grief like this:

> Clearly, issues associated with disenfranchisement in bereavement and grief deserve attention. They indicate that social outlooks often embody a judgmental element (whether explicitly articulated or not) stemming

from a society's determination to act on specific values or principles at the expense of an interest in the welfare of each of its members. In this way, disenfranchisement marginalizes, or views as negligible, the experiences of those to which it is applied. As a phenomenon deriving from specific social values or principles, disenfranchisement may be lived out in different ways in different societies or in the same society at different times. Nevertheless, those who pay even limited attention to social practices and messages easily observe disenfranchisement.[7]

Counselors who are attuned to how disenfranchisement is manifested in our society (as with the grief of racism) will be keenly aware of its presence and its effects on the lives of clients.

For clients who can benefit from understanding the disenfranchisement they have experienced and suppressed, it is important to include an appropriate level of psychoeducation about disenfranchised grief and the hidden sorrow of racism. Counselors should offer clients the opportunity to process their grief and attend to their emotions as they name and grieve racism's effects. Often, beyond the normal emotions of grief, there are more intense reactions and uniquely complicated experiences of anger, sadness, numbness, hopelessness, and depression. The erasure of Black grief, the loss, and the pain all need to be seen, heard, known, and cared about.

CASE STUDY: LATRICE'S LOSSES

Latrice came to counseling to get help with anger management. She self-described as a divorced African American female with two sons, ages four and six. She grew up in a large southeastern city with her parents and three other siblings. Latrice was seventeen years old when her father died from gunshot wounds inflicted by police officers during a routine traffic stop. The two White police officers involved in the shooting said her father resisted and became "nervous and belligerent" when the officers told him they needed to see his driver's license and vehicle registration. When he reached for "something" in the car, they opened fire and fatally wounded him. Latrice says the police report of what happened on that night seventeen years ago was vague and confusing. The police were not equipped with body cameras at that time, and the officers faced no charges.

Having unexpectedly lost the family's primary wage-earner, Latrice and her family ceased to have the income that had supported their middle-class lifestyle. A few months later, Latrice's older sister was arrested for shoplifting at a local grocery store. She entered a guilty plea and explained that she wanted to get food for her mom and younger siblings, but she did not have enough money. Although a shoplifting offense carries a typical sentence of probation and fines or a few months in jail, the judge sentenced Latrice's sister to twenty-four months of imprisonment. In jail, her sister got into a fight with some other women, resulting in a debilitating traumatic brain injury that left her permanently disabled.

Latrice gave up her dream of going to college, passing up a full four-year scholarship so she could get a job to help her mother and younger siblings in the absence of her father and older sister. Latrice is now thirty-four years old and struggling to manage her anger, especially with her two sons. She says that the smallest things they do seem to set her off. Latrice tells her counselor that she really wants to get her anger under control.

Racial injustice is woven throughout her father's death and her sister's sentencing. Latrice's pursuit of her college dream was set aside because of those events, and her sister lost her capacity to live a full life. It was more sadness than Latrice could leave behind. A previous counselor had talked to her about adverse childhood experiences and complex PTSD to explain her anger. Latrice says she did anger management work with that therapist, but they did not talk about her losses.

Latrice's new counselor introduces the concept of disenfranchised grief and asks Latrice if that resonates with her. The therapist explains that disenfranchised grief might be looming and suggests to Latrice that her anger might be a product of ambiguous loss and chronic sorrow. She asks Latrice if she thinks it would be helpful to explore her grief rather than invest time in more anger management interventions and Latrice readily agrees.

Together, they explore her father's death, her sister's incarceration, the loss of her sister's vibrancy and capacity, and her sacrificed college dreams as issues laden with grief and loss for which she didn't have any social support. Latrice says her family got some support from their community and friends when her dad died, "but I lost my sister twice: once to the incarceration and then to her disability, but no one cared." She adds, "I lost my own self—my vision for a future—when I gave up my scholarship, but nobody cared about that either. I was just another Black girl with a failed dream, and that pissed me off! I could have been so much more! I *should* have been so much more!"

Latrice and the counselor talk openly about the ways that racial bias and discrimination affected all those situations. The therapist gives Latrice a safe place to talk and to grieve each week. There is a catharsis in sharing her grief, and within six months Latrice has stopped having angry outbursts with her sons.

The first counselor focused on symptoms (anger) and behavior (outbursts). Those were not the best targets, although many counselors would have taken the same approach. Anger management work was not needed when Latrice was able to openly admit and process her ambiguous losses and disenfranchised grief.

HEARING THE CLIENT'S WHOLE STORY

The grief of racism has physical, emotional, psychological, relational, and spiritual implications. In order to recognize the disenfranchised grief of racism, counselors must be sensitive to the many ripple effects of bias, discrimination, and racism within a client's life. This requires listening to each client's whole story. It is never enough to listen only to the presenting symptoms of Black clients. Depression symptoms, relational problems, financial constraints, and health challenges do not stand alone. The stories—including the grief—of racialized groups have been historically silenced, but counselors are in a unique position to hear those stories and respond with cultural humility, empathy, and advocacy.

NOTES

1. LaVerne Hanes Collins, "Sorrow Buried Alive: Exploring the Grief of Racism," *Counseling Today* 64, no. 8 (February 2022), 13.

2. Kenneth Doka, *Disenfranchised Grief: Recognizing Hidden Sorrow* (New York: Lexington Books, 1989).

3. *Vocabulary.com*, s.v. "Disenfranchised," accessed April 7, 2023, https://www
.vocabulary.com/dictionary/disenfranchised#:~:text=The%20Old%20French%20word
%20enfranchir,their%20basic%20rights%20and%20freedom.

4. Charles A Corr, "Revisiting the Concept of Disenfranchised Grief," in *Disenfranchised Grief: New Directions, Challenges, and Strategies for Practice*, ed. Kenneth J. Doka
(Champaign, IL: Research Press, 2002), 42. This citation applies to the entire paragraph.

5. Doka, *Disenfranchised Grief.*

6. Collins, "Sorrow Buried Alive," 13.

7. Corr, "Revisiting the Concept," 42.

Part V

Overlooked Strengths

CHAPTER 11

Cultural Assets in Black Families

[W]e do not view the [Black] family as a causal Nexus in a tangle of pathology which feeds on itself. . . . It is, in our view, an absorbing, adaptive, and amazingly resilient mechanism for the socialization of its children and the civilization of its society.

—ANDREW BILLINGSLEY

THE BEST CLINICAL INTERVENTIONS FOCUS ON A PERSON'S STRENGTHS and resources, both internal and external. When challenges arise, the counselor acknowledges and validates the issues and problems, but then helps to identify and highlight the client's strengths. Attentiveness to the strengths of Black family and culture is a relatively new area of study in the counseling literature. For years, most scholarly examinations of Black families focused on indicators of weakness and instability.

Over the last fifty years, however, more has been written about the Black experience than ever before. There has been a flood of literature and research about the significance of strengths-based work with Black clients, but multicultural and diversity learning experiences in counselor education still have not typically focused on Black strengths. As a result, counselors are often only prepared to pathologize Black clients, which is more disempowering than empowering for Black families and adds to their general distrust of mental health providers.

Instead of focusing on strengths, there is a systemic tendency to adopt either a monocultural or a deficit-focused approach to Black individuals and families in counseling. The monocultural approach assumes a high level of sameness for all clients, and overlooks the strengths held in diverse family scenarios. A deficit-focused approach to Black lifestyles suggests there is a greater degree of pathology in Black families than in White families.[1]

Both of those approaches portray White American standards as the measurement of health and normalcy. Neither of those approaches show an appropriate regard for historical and experiential differences between Black and White Americans.

DEFINITION OF FAMILY

Merriam-Webster defines "nuclear family" as the core members of a family.[2] Nuclear is associated with "nucleus," meaning "something essential." It is generally accepted that a nuclear family consists only of people connected by partnership and parenthood, as in a set of parents and their children.

It is not uncommon for Black families to define family more broadly than *Merriam-Webster* does. So, to be most effective with members of Black families, counselors must understand the concept of family in a manner inclusive of Black cultural norms. Child Trends, a Maryland-based research organization, offers this definition of Black family: "a group of at least one self-identified Black adult related by birth, marriage, adoption, or choice to one or more children (infancy through adolescence). The adult(s) may also be residing with or economically, socially, and emotionally responsible for the child(ren)'s well-being."[3] The strength of this inclusive definition is in its flexibility, wherein the portals of family entry include birth, marriage, adoption, *or choice.*

By the dictionary definition, African slaves were already excluded from the "essential" configuration because in Southern states slaves were forbidden to legally marry. Western society elevated the patriarchal nuclear family as being the ideal model, then denied that model to those they wanted to oppress. The marriage ceremony for enslaved people involved the couple jumping over a broomstick as a sign of their covenant, but the marriage was not legally recognized. Their union and their children were disregarded whenever slaveholders chose to divide families either for profit or for punishment. People in slavery knew they were seen as a commodity. As long as they were enslaved, they lacked any control over their family configurations.

Western society elevated the patriarchal nuclear family as being the ideal model, then denied that model to those they wanted to oppress.

Culturally sensitive concepts of family will allow family members' needs—rather than the nuclear definition—to determine the configuration of their "essential members." Family configurations in Africa were always broader than the "two parents plus children" idea of nuclear. People of African descent used their native extended family conceptualization as their model for mutual emotional, relational, and economic support, all without bloodline restrictions. Moms, dads, aunties, uncles, brothers, sisters, pap-paps, nanas, and cousins were relational *roles* that were not always genealogically based. The only "essential" family unit was one wherein the people experienced love and care.

When a monocultural nuclear family model is seen as the standard or the ideal, the variety of family structures within Black American cultures can be devalued or even viewed with disdain. Traditional theories applied to White families draw conclusions of inherent weakness and inferiority about Black family structures. Statistical representations have frequently and strategically portrayed Black family life as dysfunctional, crumbling, and unstable. The implied messages are that Black families have more pathology than White families and that Black people do not manage family life responsibly. If integrated into a Black person's way of thinking, the "weak state" message of the Black family adds another log to the fire of internalized self-defeat. On the other hand, it adds another log to a subtly burning sense of superiority for Whites. Neither of these fiery biases is easily extinguished.

Bias is insidious. Black clients themselves can unwittingly buy into the "weak family structure" narrative. Even clinicians who have confidence in their objectivity may fail to see the Black family unit or the extended family as a strength for a client of African descent. As such, the problem/deficit focus is maintained and a positive/strengths-based focus is cast aside. With the management of bias—or ideally in the absence of it—the counselor can accept that adequate family functioning does not follow a single and exclusive model and can be manifested in multiple ways. A solely pathological focus on Black families serves to reinforce America's social hierarchy and to blame the victim.

A HISTORY OF PATHOLOGICAL CHARACTERIZATIONS

Factors that influence Black adaptive functioning are frequently pathologized. In turn, important strengths are dismissed as deviant or unhealthy. One historical example of this pathologizing is the Moynihan Report of 1965. While serving as Assistant Secretary for the Department of Labor, Daniel Patrick Moynihan published a report titled "The Negro Family: The Case for National Action." Moynihan was a sociologist who became a New York state politician and eventually served twenty-four years as a Democratic US Senator. The Moynihan Report called upon the federal government for "a new kind of national goal: the establishment of a stable Negro family structure."[4]

Moynihan spoke of the Black family as "crumbling" in urban areas. He saw the Black family as the problem with educational attainment gaps. Moynihan pointed to (a) "illegitimate" births in African American homes, (b) an African American divorce rate that was 1.5 percent higher than that of Whites, and (c) a resulting increase in women as heads of African American households.

Moynihan recognized the damage and the hardship put upon African Americans by the US political and financial systems (e.g., slavery, failed reconstruction, wage gaps, and other inequities). However, his deficit-based perspectives on Black America set up one particular configuration and family model as the standard for all families. He believed that there was "much evidence that a considerable number of Negro families have managed to break out of *the tangle of pathology* and to establish themselves as stable, effective units, *living according to patterns of American society in general*"[5] (emphasis added). This was just one of many points in the Moynihan Report that caused a storm of controversy. Homes headed by African American single mothers are not inherently pathological, and that label is an unjust characterization. Competent single parents lead healthy homes everywhere. In many cases, their families are made even stronger by extended family or other support systems.[6]

Any deficit-based perspective "limits psychological science by overlooking the broader experiences, value, perspectives, and strengths that individuals who face systemic marginalization often bring to their societies."[7] Counselors must reject assumptions that a minoritized or racialized identity is a deficit. Research has consistently demonstrated that a person's identity as a member of a marginalized group is often the source of strengths that may help them succeed.[8]

Even after acknowledging a range of historical injustices against African Americans, the Moynihan Report perpetuated a victim-blaming mentality and suggested that the task at hand was a campaign to "fix" Black families, rather than a campaign for systemic transformation and taking a stand against racism, bias, housing discrimination, or unjust policies where the real pathologies reside. Advocacy for systemic change would have provided a more respectful approach to the effects of discrimination. Today, the Moynihan Report still influences American thought. Counselors must resist the Moynihan mindset and give corrective attention to any tendency to pathologize client experiences that are different from their own. This is a critical task toward dismantling deficiency models imposed upon African American and other Black communities.

DISMANTLING DEFICIENCY MODELS

The totality of Black family strength is too broad for an exhaustive examination within the scope of this work, so I have chosen to provide a high-level look at one preeminent seminal work and one recent study related to the cultural strengths of Black family values and lifestyles. At different points in history, these studies shed light on Black cultural values and traditions that are often misunderstood for the strength they offer, the history they carry, the value they bring to life, and the survival they inspire.

Five Historical Core Strengths

Counselors must identify family strengths in a culturally unbiased way. To be sure, a strength in one situation could certainly present itself as a weakness in another situation. Conversely, however, a weakness in one scenario can be a strength in a different context or when a different set of measurement criteria are applied.[9] Robert Hill made this point in his seminal 1972 book titled *The Strengths of Black Families*. Hill was one of several researchers who began turning attention to the strengths of Black family lifestyles in the 1960s and 1970s[10] defining family strengths as "those traits which facilitate the ability of the family to meet the needs of its members and the demands made upon it by systems outside the family unit."[11]

Hill's definition facilitates a culturally unbiased understanding of familial strength for any culture. Using census data and other information, he documented five characteristic Black family strengths: (1) strong kinship bonds, (2) strong work orientation, (3) adaptability of family roles, (4) strong achievement orientation, and (5) strong religious orientation.[12] He sought to demonstrate that stability and strength, rather than instability and weakness, are the model patterns for both low- and middle-income Black families. These traits can also be present in families of other races and cultures, but they manifest uniquely or in greater proportion in the Black experience.

Strong Kinship Bonds

Whether African American, Afro-Caribbean, or African immigrant, the people of African descent in America all share a native cultural legacy where family life is highly valued, and the definition of family goes beyond the expected genealogical limits of some other cultures. Culturally responsive counselors honor that legacy and build upon those cultural strengths. Any strengths-based approach to problem-solving with a Black client needs to consider biological and non-biological family members as resources that can often be definitively addressed as cultural strengths and therapeutic assets.

Informal adoption and kinship care are mainstays in Black life.[13] Children sold on an auction block without their parents or siblings found new loving family members among the people joined with them in slavery. Women and men sold downriver to strangers needed—and found—people to call family. It was a system of reciprocity: Slaves paid it forward and cared for people they did not know because they hoped the same care would be extended to them and their own family members in due time. It was simply the right thing to do. And it worked! It still works! Families are broadly defined in Black cultures, based on relational roles, and everyone is better for it. If you interact like a sister, you *are* my sister. If you interact like an auntie, you *are* my auntie. If you do for me what dads do for their children, you *are* my dad. And so on and so forth.

Kinship extension practices also have an important role in the support networks of African Americans and other people of African descent. The term "fictive kin" is commonly used to refer to people who are regarded as family but are not related by blood or by marriage.[14] Research has shown that these relationships operate as a means to strengthen family and not merely as a substitute for family deficits.[15]

This model of care and support is indicative of the strength of community care and non-kinship bonds in Black American life. This community model has been positioned by ethnocentric others to be a deficit model, a deviant model—but it is in fact a brilliant model. It did not come about because of slavery. It was an existing African model used during slavery.

Hill described kinship patterns that he called "the absorption of individuals," "the absorption of families," and "informal adoption."[16] This heritage of wider essential family systems served Africans well in their motherland, served African Americans well through chattel slavery and segregation, and continues to serve African Americans and other Blacks well today.

The absorption of individuals specifically includes the elderly and minor children born to single parents.[17] Using census data, Hill found that the likelihood of Black families taking in young relatives was much greater than the chances of White families doing the same.[18]

Hill's research also noted that "doubling up," or joining multiple families together in a supportive unit, is a common practice, especially when new families move into urban areas.[19] This "absorption of families" has been a regular occurrence among Black families since chattel slavery.

The third manifestation of kinship bonds in Black families is "informal adoption," or the taking-in of children by Black families on an informal or unofficial basis. Hill noted that Black families have an annual informal "adoption" rate more than ten times greater than that of formal adoption agencies.[20]

Counselors do their clients a disservice by assuming that a culturally normative family structure for Black families is burdensome and needs to be fixed or even pitied. The bond of supportive kinship is a protective factor for racialized and minoritized communities. As a result of these strong kinship ties, many African American and other Black families grow into extended families in which relatives with diverse bloodlines integrate into a network of mutual psychosocial and economic support. This is one of the most important considerations that proponents of the deficit-based perspective overlook in their assessment of Black families.

Strong Work Orientation

Hill's research pointed to the strong emphasis on work and self-help that are highly valued in most Black families. This has been sorely misunderstood by social scientists, who have often looked at rates of unemployment or public assistance and cast blame on the victim, rather than the discriminatory systems that work against them. Hill also pointed to the dual-income structure of Black families.[21] It was common for women in Black families to work outside the home long before working women became the norm in the United States. At the time of Hill's original research, approximately two-thirds of the wives in Black families were employed outside the home, compared to about half of the wives in White families.[22] This strong emphasis on work in low- and middle-income African American families, which is the norm, is frequently overlooked.

Adaptability of Family Roles

Hill's research revealed that the normal pattern of decisions among Black households was equalitarian rather than matriarchal, as had been suggested in previous literature.[23] Black men were shown to be highly involved in both decision making and domestic responsibilities. The flexibility in African American families was likely due in part to economic necessity, as women and even adolescents often work to help support the family. As a result, household tasks are also carried out with more role versatility. Without stereotypical gender expectations, Black families have the ability to more easily manage changing circumstances, and Hill identifies this flexibility as a specific source of stability and strength in Black families.[24]

Strong Achievement Orientation

For higher education and achievement orientation, Hill noted that higher proportions of Black students cited parental pressure to finish college compared to White students.[25] He found that Blacks from lower-income, single-parent homes reported higher occupational aspirations than Whites from lower-income, two-parent homes: "The salience of strong achievement orientation in Black families is often unrecognized by Whites who do not see this exhibited according to their own cultural expectations."[26] When talking to their children, Black families tend to place a strong emphasis on ambition, believing in yourself and that you can do anything, and envisioning your future beyond any confinements in your present situation. Education is seen as the gateway to advancement and upward mobility. Hill referred to this culture of determination and aspiration as "one of the unheralded strengths of Blacks."[27]

Strong Religious Orientation

This strength refers to the role of one's faith and belief in a "transcendent being" (God) or "higher power." Historically, the reliance on religion and spirituality in Black culture has been larger than life itself—indeed, faith has been a source of strength and a key to Black survival.[28] Black theology speaks hope for today and for eternity, when everything else in life is clouded by adversity and insecurity. Faith has been the center of the redemptive message, not just from an after-life perspective, but for navigating life's daily struggles. As we understand trauma definitions today, many Black lives have been saturated with racial trauma, and many have found healing from the past and hope for the future in their personal faith. The institution of the historically Black Church and its role as a strength for Black individuals will be explored in the next chapter.

Updated Findings for Black Family Strength

Hill's work provided a snapshot of Black life on the heels of the Civil Rights Movement, a time when the nation's attention was directed to the social and economic position of Black Americans. Over the fifty years since the initial publication of his findings, much has been written about the strengths of Black families. What does this look like in modern times and contemporary terms? A study published by Child Trends in 2022 set out to offer a new and more nuanced understanding of Black family life in recent years.[29]

Child Trends' findings are largely consistent with the cultural strengths that Robert Hill investigated as key protective characteristics for Black families. The Child Trends study labels these shared cultural values, traditions, and practices as "cultural assets" that have nourished and nurtured families over time.[30]

From Hill's findings in 1972 to the Child Trends study in 2022, the categories of identified strengths have varied only slightly. The cultural assets echoed in 2022 are extended kin and social networks, religiosity and spirituality, and role flexibility. To those three assets originally recognized in Hill's work, the Child Trends study adds optimism, which shares some similar characteristics with the educational and achievement categories in Hill's book.

Optimism

Child Trends defines optimism as "the penetrating belief held by most Black families that conditions will improve."[31] Child Trends cites studies showing that even through situational or economic adversities, a sense of optimism about the future is an asset for Black families today, and this holds true across socioeconomic strata.[32] Research shows that optimism is associated with better mental and physical health outcomes for Black Americans, but the mechanisms behind this connection are not clearly understood. Prior to the COVID-19 pandemic of 2020 to 2022, Black people had made progress—although slowly—in education and health, which improved their quality of life in comparison to earlier generations. These advancements, together with optimistic beliefs as an asset, appear to be contributing factors to positive outcomes. The other strengths serve much the same functions as described in 1972.

Extended Kin and Social Networks

Family continues to involve both biological and non-biological kin. These ties still play a beneficial role in Black families, including through support and resources in response to unexpected crises and care for vulnerable loved ones. Counselors who discourage Black family members from these practices or advocate for "firmer boundaries" may be undermining exchanges that contribute to Black families' psychological well-being and survival in racist and unjust environments. A counselor's individualistic values may be in conflict with the collectivistic values of community survival. For example, to suggest that a client is enabling or fostering dependence by financially supporting biological or voluntary kin shows a disregard for a family strength and cultural asset. Counselors must not impose their "self-first" values onto a culture that has survived systemic racism, economic hardship, and hostile environments by sharing resources with others. Clients need to know that counselors respect those decisions and can empathize without judgment when the client opens their home, sacrifices their resources, or sets aside their own wealth accumulation for the good of someone else. Through one lens this is a sacrifice, but through another it is community survival.

Role Flexibility

Role flexibility continues to operate as a strength by enabling families to navigate fluidly without gender and role restrictions. As needs arise, family members adapt and may assume responsibilities that do not necessarily fit age or gender expectations. Counselors must refrain from any suggestion that a family's role flexibility is pathological or invalid. Encouraging a client to "speak up for themselves" or "set better boundaries" when that is not the client's desire shows a cultural disregard for the way family members and voluntary kin help one another respond to changing circumstances. For example, suggesting to a grandparent that they invest in living their best life rather than being available for unexpected care of their grandchildren may create unforeseen cognitive discrepancy and do more harm than good for the client's family system.

Religiosity and Spirituality

Religion and spirituality still play important roles as cultural assets in the lives of Black people. Child Trends reports that 74 percent of Black people in the United States report a deep belief in God.[33] Many also state that regular prayer is important to them. It is notable that age and immigration status account for some interesting differences. For example, younger Black people report less religious involvement than older generations. Additionally, Sub-Saharan African immigrants and Afro-Caribbean immigrants are more likely to practice orthodox Christian religions or Islam than African Americans. Most Black people in America attend a Black church, and 66 percent identify as Protestants. Black people say the church has been significant in their lives on many levels, including spiritual uplift, community building, and economic advancement.

Differences Based on Socioeconomic Experiences

An important addition to the understanding of how Black families navigate life is in the addition of intra-race comparisons that consider distinctions in varied socioeconomic experiences. With this perspective, income and social standing can be used to draw distinctions in family structure and practices. Research also notes that "even within-group examinations of Black families that attend to historical and structural issues within U.S. systems tend to underscore White middle-class standards as aspirational."[34]

The Child Trends study acknowledges that within-group experiential differences are not mutually exclusive from either the Moynihan deficit-based perspective of instability and pathology or Hill's counter-focus on family strengths.[35]

Managing Ethnocentrism

Ethnocentrism, or seeing one's own ethnoracial experience as superior, limits a counselor's ability to objectively attend to the shared values and practices of Black family life. Counselors must avoid devaluing attributes that have served Black families well for centuries. Allow clients to explain *why* and *how* extended kinship and flexible roles work for them. Listen without judgment to the problems that are solved. Avoid pathologizing. Engage with clients from a place of cultural humility and learn. In this way, clients are empowered to use their cultural assets, and a better counselor is in the room.

NOTES

1. David D. Royse and Gladys T. Turner, "Strengths of Black Families: A Black Community's Perspective," *Social Work* 25, no. 5 (September 1980): 407–40, https://doi.org/10.1093/sw/25.5.407.

2. "Why Is It Called the Nuclear Family?" Merriam-Webster.com, accessed April 9, 2023, https://www.merriam-webster.com/words-at-play/nuclear-family-history-origin.

3. Christina M. Lloyd et al., "Reimagining Black Families' Cultural Assets Can Inform Policies and Practices That Enhance Their Well-Being," Child Trends, February 22, 2022, https://www.childtrends.org/publications/reimagining-black-families-cultural-assets-can-inform-policies-and-practices-that-enhance-their-well-being.

4. Daniel Patrick Moynihan, *The Negro Family: The Case for National Action* (Washington, DC.: U.S. Department of Labor, 1965), 29.

5. Moynihan, *The Negro Family*.

6. Nancy Boyd-Franklin, *Black Families in Therapy: Understanding the African American Experience* (New York: Guilford Press, 2003), 19; Marion Lindblad-Goldberg, Joyce Lynn Dukes, and John H. Lasley, "Stress in Black, Low-Income, Single-Parent Families: Normative and Dysfunctional Patterns," *American Journal of Orthopsychiatry* 58, no. 1 (February 1988): 104–20, https://doi.org/10.1111/j.1939-0025.1988.tb01570.x.

7. David M. Silverman et al., "The Ongoing Development of Strength-Based Approaches to People Who Hold Systemically Marginalized Identities," *Personality and Social Psychology Review* 27, no. 3 (January 12, 2023): 255–71, https://doi.org/10.1177/10888683221145243.

8. Silverman et al., "The Ongoing Development."

9. Robert Bernard Hill, *The Strengths of Black Families* (Lanham, MD: University Press of America, 2003), xix.

10. Boyd-Franklin, *Black Families in Therapy*.

11. Hill, *The Strengths of Black Families*, xix.

12. Hill, *The Strengths of Black Families*, xi–xx.

13. Sojourner Ahébée, "How Informal Adoptions Became a Mainstay of African American Family Life," WHYY (January 14, 2022), https://whyy.org/segments/how-informal-adoptions-became-a-mainstay-of-african-american-family-life.

14. Carol B. Stack, *All Our Kin: Strategies for Survival in a Black Community* (New York, NY: Harper & Row, 1974); Robert Taylor et al., "Fictive Kin Networks among African Americans, Black Caribbeans, and Non-Latino Whites," *Journal of Family Issues* 43, no. 1 (February 19, 2021): 20–46, https://doi.org/10.1177/0192513X21993188.

15. Taylor et al., "Fictive Kin Networks," 20–46.

16. Silverman, et al, "The Ongoing Development."

17. Hill, *The Strengths of Black Families*, 1.

18. Hill, *The Strengths of Black Families*, 3.

19. Hill, *The Strengths of Black Families*, 2.

20. Hill, *The Strengths of Black Families*, 3.

21. Hill, *The Strengths of Black Families*, 7.

22. Hill, *The Strengths of Black Families*, 7.

23. Hill, *The Strengths of Black Families*, 12.

24. Hill, *The Strengths of Black Families*, 11.

25. Hill, *The Strengths of Black Families*, 24.

26. Boyd-Franklin, *Black Families in Therapy*, 21.

27. Hill, *The Strengths of Black Families*, 21.

28. Hill, *The Strengths of Black Families*, 27.

29. Lloyd et al., "Reimagining Black Families' Cultural Assets."

30. Andrew Billingsley, *Climbing Jacob's Ladder: The Enduring Legacy of African-American Families* (New York: Simon & Schuster, 1994); Hill, *The Strengths of Black Families*; Stack, *All Our Kin*; Lloyd et al., "Reimagining Black Families' Cultural Assets."

31. Lloyd et al., "Reimagining Black Families' Cultural Assets," section 3, paragraph 7.

32. Lloyd et al., "Reimagining Black Families' Cultural Assets," section 3, paragraph 7.

33. Jeff Diamant, "Three-Quarters of Black Americans Believe in God of the Bible or Other Holy Scripture" (Pew Research Center, January 31, 2022), https://www.pewresearch.org/fact-tank/2021/03/24/three-quarters-of-black-americans-believe-in-god-of-the-bible-or-other-holy-scripture.

34. Lloyd et al., "Reimagining Black Families' Cultural Assets."

35. Lloyd et al., "Reimagining Black Families' Cultural Assets."

CHAPTER 12

This Far by Faith

Religion and Spirituality in Black Life

I found that I knew not only that there was a God but that I was a child of God.
When I understood that, when I comprehended that, more than that, when I internalized that, ingested that, I became courageous.

—Maya Angelou

"We've come this far by faith, leaning on the Lord. Trusting in His holy word. He's never failed me yet. Ohhhh! Oh-Oh-Oh! Oh-Oh-Oh! Can't turn around. We've come this far by faith."[1] "We've Come This Far by Faith," written in 1956 by Albert Goodson, is one of the most classic and time-honored gospel songs ever to be rendered in the historically Black Church. By the 1960s, it was popular in congregations across the country because:

> In a manner similar to many of the Old Testament lament psalms, this text affirms God's saving power in the past; God's compassion and providential care for his people throughout history give us hope for the future. Thus the text becomes a marker or milestone on life's journey: "We've come this far by faith, leaning on the Lord" (1 Sam. 7:12, "Thus far has the Lord helped us"). With confidence in the Lord's help we can go forward and face "burdens . . . misery and strife."[2]

The song captures the essence of Black Protestant theology and social determination. The lyrics provide a powerful refrain about the resilience of The Black Church as a people and as an institution.

Strong Religious Beliefs and Practices

In 2020, 72 percent of Black Americans identified as Christian. More than six in ten (63 percent) are Protestant, of which 35 percent identify as evangelical and 28 percent identify as non-evangelical Protestants. Seven percent of Black Americans are Catholic, while two percent are Muslims and two percent are Buddhists. Two percent are another religion, and one percent identify as Jehovah's Witnesses; less than one percent identify as Latter-day Saint, Orthodox Christian, Jewish, or Hindu. A little more than one in five Black Americans (21 percent) are religiously unaffiliated.[3]

In the Pew Research Center's Religious Landscape Study, it was notable that when compared to White, Latino, Asian and Other/Mixed racial and ethnic groups, Black respondents led in the percentage of people who reported:[4]

- Believing in God, with absolute certainty
- Religion is very important in their life
- Attending religious services at least once per week
- Praying at least daily
- Participating in prayer, scripture study, or religious education groups at least once a week
- Meditating at least once per week
- Feeling spiritual peace and wellbeing at least once per week
- Looking to religion as a source of guidance on right and wrong (compared to looking to philosophy/reason, common sense, science, or not knowing where they look for guidance on right/ wrong)
- Reading Scripture at least once per week

- Interpreting scripture as the Word of God that should be taken literally
- Believing in heaven
- Believing in hell

The Pew study is consistent with previous findings that African Americans exhibit higher levels of religious participation than do Whites.[5] The 63 percent of Black Americans who identify as Protestant create a unique social institution known as The Black Church.

THE BLACK CHURCH AS AN INSTITUTION
There is no social institution in the Black community as multidimensional as The Black Church, a collective institution comprising the totality of the historically and predominantly African American Christian Protestant congregations in the United States. Any African American congregation adhering to Christian teaching may be referred to as "a" Black church, but the term "*The* Black Church" signifies a general and collective description of Black religious heritage. While The Black Church is larger than a single congregation or denomination, there are certain cultural elements that carry across these faith communities.

"The Black Church" was originally a scholarly term, but it is now a culturally accepted expression that includes the African Methodist Episcopal (A.M.E.) Church, the African Methodist Episcopal Zion Church (A.M.E. Zion), the Christian Methodist Episcopal (C.M.E.) Church, the National Baptist Convention (N.B.C.), the National Baptist Convention of America (N.B.C.A.), the Progressive National Convention (P.N.C.), the Church of God in Christ (COGIC), some Southern Missionary Baptists, and the largely African American nondenominational churches founded by African Americans and known for Black worship styles.[6] More than half of all African American individuals in the United States (53 percent at the turn of the millennium) identified as attending one of these churches.[7] Black religion in America has been most strongly influenced by Baptist and Methodist traditions, with characteristic emotional expression and spontaneity.[8]

In 1903, W. E. B. Du Bois released a sociological study under the title "The Negro Church," the source from which the name "The Black Church" evolved. Du Bois described the Negro Church as the sole African-born social institution to survive the transatlantic slave trade. Du Bois stated that the leadership of the Negro Church had simply been shifted from the African priest or medicine man to the Christian preacher in America. The Negro Church preserved aspects of African tribal culture and became the social hub of the community. Du Bois believed that the slave church was African rather than Christian. Du Bois described church congregations as the true units of Black American life and community, both dividing and defining the race.[9]

THE LOCAL BLACK CHURCH AS A LOCAL TRIBE

I recall listening to my mom and dad at the dinner table when I was a child. They knew people by the local church they attended. My mom would mention a family acquaintance by name, and my dad would use that person's church as an identifier. He would say, "Oh, yeah, she goes to Emmanuel [Baptist Church]." Or if he wasn't sure, his response might be, "Do you mean Mary from Second Baptist?" It was amazing to me how the identities of local people were tied to the name of their church. After all these years, I still find myself using church affiliation as a reference point.

African cultures identified people by their tribal subgroup, such as Ewe, Akan, or Ashanti in Ghana. Here, my parents used a person's church to identify them. In a small-town environment, a person could easily have been identified by the street they lived on, but instead were known by the church they attended. Just as each tribe in an African context has its own cultural traditions, each church congregation has its own "personality." The local churches were generally composed of family groupings, but some were known to attract the middle class while others attracted the working or non-working poor. Some worshipped with more emotionality and spontaneity as the norm, while others followed a more prescribed and predictable order of service.

Research conducted by the Pew Research Center found that African Americans report religion having a greater influence on them than on people of other races. Compared to other racial groups, African Americans have a higher percentage of people who say that they believe in God with complete conviction (83 percent); that religion is very important to them (75 percent); that they pray daily (73 percent); or that they attend religious services at least once a week (47 percent).[10]

The Black Church has always been more than just the epicenter of spiritual life. Understanding how The Black Church provides more than a worship center requires insight into the many cultural, psychological, economic, political, and community benefits delivered directly by The Black Church.

The Black Church has long served as the backbone of African American communities and the heartbeat of social integration. For Black communities, The Black Church was the first social hall, led the first voter registration drives, was the home of the first Sunday buffet, and was the first institution that offered interest-free loans to Black members when hard times struck. Informally speaking, The Black Church was also the first counseling center in the Black community. Their chosen counselor was—and often still is—the pastor.

Today, scientific research abounds regarding mental wellness and illness, brain function, addictions, and treatment interventions. Despite this knowledge, disparities still exist in the availability and quality of professional care in Black communities. In these communities, mental illness was frequently misunderstood, addiction frequently normalized, and treatment frequently stigmatized, so people more often sought solutions from spiritual practices or advice from a pastor rather than seeking professional mental health care. The historical background of slavery and the Back Church explains this cultural pattern.

CULTURAL CARRYOVERS

In Africa, mental health and spirituality have always been closely related, but the subject of mental health is largely taboo because the suffering person and their entire family are seen as cursed.[11] African people have historically viewed such disturbances as evidence of an external attack, such as a spell, a bewitching, or the presence of an evil spirit. African cultures also tend to view hereditary problems as generational curses—entire families become stigmatized, and the family's women and girls become marked as un-marriable for fear of them passing down the curse to their descendants.

To match these metaphysical explanations for their troubles, Africans sought metaphysical remedies, usually from traditional healers or priests who would perform ceremonies, cast out demons, and reverse the curses that plagued the afflicted. As Samir Abi observed, "the success of religious practices has not been scientifically proven, but it is obvious that belief in divine powers can lead to recovery."[12]

Historically, some denominations in The Black Church have also treated mental health issues as taboo or metaphysical, and their response to the Western model of mental illness is frequently a spiritual response. Centuries upon centuries later, the pastor has replaced the tribal healer as the person to whom one would take their problems, thus confirming the aforementioned statement by W. E. B. Du Bois that the role of the African priest or medicine man was conveyed to the Christian preacher in America during the era of chattel slavery.

Plantation owners generally set strict limitations on the number of enslaved people allowed to congregate without the observation of an overseer, so slaves longing for the chance to gather began to meet in secret. Often called "the invisible church," these gatherings provided a much-needed psychological and emotional release. Slaves attended these gatherings in the belief that they would one day have a better life, either on earth or in heaven.

These slaves were able to listen to the Bible without the twisted interpretation of scripture provided by their oppressors, and they came to recognize that equality, freedom, and dignity were not above them—exactly what the plantation owners feared would happen. In many cases, the leaders of these secret congregations were formerly enslaved people who had achieved at least a basic level of reading ability. Because of the freedom and literacy they had attained, slaves held these preachers in the highest regard and placed a great deal of faith in them, looking to them not just for spiritual direction but also for general guidance, knowledge about the Underground Railroad, and assistance in reading or interpreting written papers. A preacher became the go-to person for the common problems of life.

Preachers within The Black Church have continued in that elevated standing over the years, maintaining their role as the advisor or "go-to person" for guidance, counsel, and prayer on issues ranging from marriage and parenting to finances and mental distress.

MENTAL HEALTH AND SPIRITUAL HEALTH AS SYNONYMOUS

The Black Church still operates to address more than spiritual life. By necessity, the Church seeks overall improvement in quality of life by addressing the biopsychosocial and spiritual needs of its community, serving as the spiritual emergency room for every kind of life malady. Historically, even psychological health has been addressed purely as a spiritual function instead of a biological function. With that approach, good spiritual health is good mental health. In the past, this belief has discredited the possibility of seeking professional help for depression, anxiety, stress management, marriage, parenting, and other problems, implying that these issues were signs of a spiritual deficit that could be remedied with spiritual practices alone.

Drawing on Faith for Strength

Many people in The Black Church view mental health and spiritual health as synonymous. A strong relationship with God has been viewed as the answer to depression, anxiety, loneliness, and other problems. With these beliefs, the abstract concepts of mind, soul, and spirit become unconsciously and inseparably interwoven with—or even override—the physical concept of the human brain. The mind is subsequently treated as spiritual, without regard for the brain as a physical organ. When mental health becomes synonymous with spiritual health, a person draws on their faith for strength.

That strength has always been necessary for survival; it is a strength that is *expected* in the Black community. Where else was a person to turn in the midst of chattel slavery, Jim Crow segregation, and systemic racism—except to their faith? Messages of hope carried them: "Give it to the Lord." "God won't give you more than you can bear." "Just trust Him." "Let the Lord fight your battles." If oppressed Black people could do nothing else, they could come to church every week and pray, cry, scream, jump, dance, and feel so much better with that release! It was indeed a remedy, an answer, a relief. Seven days later, they would return for another dose.

> Minoritized people hear subtle daily messages that their life and preferences—particularly those of a spiritual nature—are undesirable, odd, or abnormal.

In the contemporary Black Church, leaders are giving more attention to mental health and are now integrating messages that encourage professional help-seeking. The pastors' long-standing influence allows them to play an important role in raising mental health awareness. More and more, churches in Black communities are engaging in mental wellness and social service programs. Pastors are making more referrals to community- and faith-based programs in deference to the expertise of trained mental health professionals, and counselors are collaborating with churches to provide services to members.

RELIGION AS TREATMENT BARRIER OR PROVIDER BIAS

When developing client case conceptualizations and treatment plans, one of the essential steps is the identification of hurdles and obstacles to care, sometimes known as "treatment barriers." These are variables that impede a client's ability to obtain or sustain engagement in treatment. I have heard many counselors point to clients' religious beliefs as treatment barriers and label African American and other Black clients as treatment-resistant when they choose religion or spirituality over psychotherapeutic models of care.

Statistics suggest that a huge percentage of Blacks and African Americans have unmet treatment needs. However, included among those with "unmet treatment needs" are people who, with religious or spiritual support alone, are managing life just as well as those on medication or in therapy. A person can choose to manage medical problems using lifestyle or holistic interventions and not be defined as having an unmet treatment need.

Clinicians have a responsibility to be aware of the numerous positive effects that participation in religious activities can have on a client's physical, emotional, and social well-being.[13] In general, mental health professionals tend to be secular and nonreligious, and they receive very limited, if any, training on religious diversity.[14] This lack of training may lead to prejudicial attitudes toward all aspects of religious belief and practice, which will make it difficult to work with many of their clients.[15]

If love, exercise, diet, and other lifestyle changes can affect brain function, is it impossible for spiritual practices to also affect dopamine and serotonin? Clients have a right to make autonomous decisions about how they handle life. As Ryan and Deci noted "Supporting autonomy and competence is supporting the fundamental human capabilities for living a full life."[16]

Elements of the mainstream media's news and entertainment programming reinforce stereotypes of religion and religious people as "superstitious, narrow-minded, rigid in thought or behavior, endorsing magical and fantasy over science, and (being) self-righteous about how to live one's life and make various important life decisions."[17] It is rare to see positive messages highlighting the benefits of faith or religion for mental health. This is sorely disadvantageous for members of Black communities where three-quarters of Blacks surveyed by the Pew Research Center indicated that religion is very important in their lives.[18]

Across all faiths, religious practices have been shown in scholarly research to have positive benefits on people's mental health and happiness, with both direct and indirect effects. Activities associated with religion, such as praying, reading religious texts, and participating in various kinds of worship have the potential to foster pleasant feelings and a sense of well-being, which can directly contribute to improved mental health and general well-being.[19]

Historically, there was no clear distinction between mental health and spiritual health in The Black Church.

The clinical models and frameworks from which counseling was developed have generally come from a European American perspective and lens. In the American treatment system, medical and psychotherapeutic interventions are typically thought to have greater credibility or efficacy than religious or faith-based responses. Through that lens, people of faith are viewed as being bound by psychological or sociocultural treatment barriers if they choose to manage their mental or emotional health with spiritual or cultural remedies. A culturally sensitive counselor must reject that view and realize that barriers apply to people who want treatment that is not easily accessible. For example, if an African American desires to obtain professional mental health care but lives in a remote region where the distance, transportation, and limited internet connectivity make engagement difficult, that individual has a treatment barrier that restricts their access to services. If, on the other hand, the individual has full access to mental health treatment but chooses to seek a spiritual or religious answer instead of medical or behavioral health care for their problem, it is entirely a question of beliefs and preferences.

Values are not barriers—they are choices. A counselor may disagree with a client's choices. They may have strong feelings of disapproval about a client's values. What matters, though, is the counselor's acceptance of the client's "irrevocable right and capacity of self-direction."[20] The client's autonomy must be respected without judgment. Therefore, when the autonomy of a client or potential client results in a help-seeking choice outside the counselor's realm of traditional therapy models, a counselor's bias may kick in and they may think that the client's treatment need is unmet. This is not an unmet treatment need, but a provider bias.

CULTURAL DEFICIT MODEL

Racially and ethnically diverse clients terminate psychotherapy after the first session significantly more often than other clients.[21] Even the most subtle counselor bias can cause a client to terminate services early in the process. Sue and colleagues explain that "cultural deficit models tend to view culturally diverse groups as possessing dysfunctional values and belief systems, which they often considered handicaps to be overcome and sources of shame."[22] Fundamentally, oppressed people hear subtle daily messages that their life and preferences are undesirable, odd, or abnormal.

African American and other Black clients recognize that bias and prejudices can be directly or indirectly working against them in any cross-cultural interaction. In counseling, the client may expect that the counselor will be disparaging or will deem their faith to be irrational. So the client may hesitate to disclose the depth of their religious conviction and the faith foundation that guides their life, lest the counselor attempt to question or dissuade them.

I have seen and heard of people getting as much relief (or more) from a weekly church service in the Black tradition with singing, dancing, and preaching as others get from therapeutic practices such as mindfulness, journaling, talk therapy, or even medication. Is that invariably the case? Of course not. However, a culturally relevant reponse will make room for religious practices and principles in the development of every bio-psychosocial-spiritual treatment plan.

Accurate diagnosis and medical referrals are essential here because severe and persistent mental illness (SPMI) and neurological disorders should always be treated by a medical professional. However, for more common, low-severity problems, counselors must be cautious not to impose their values on anyone who chooses religious coping approaches.

MANAGING PROVIDER BIAS

In essence, bias politely asserts, "This client needs what I offer, because the only thing I value is my school of thought. Nothing else will work as well." To provide services in an ethical manner, counselors must put themselves in the client's shoes, adopt a posture of cultural humility, and make a clear distinction between counselor prejudice and treatment barriers. Instead of seeing cultural differences in terms of therapeutic barriers, I urge counselors to examine their own implicit biases.

Every counselor has biases. Culturally sensitive counselors learn to recognize their own biases and how those biases may affect their interpretation and therapeutic judgment. They must use ongoing training and supervision to address their biases and to gain respect for what their clients value. Culturally sensitive counselors understand that to impose monocultural standards without regard for client group differences is in itself a form of oppression and therefore constitutes unethical practice.

Counselors must commit to personal and ongoing inventory of their biases. How do your preconceived notions about religious and culturally based help-seeking affect your judgment? Consider how your prejudices may get in the way of your ability to respect individuals who are different from you. Leave preconceived monocultural notions about treatment and your personal ideals about client care at the door.

African Americans and other Black clients have had their important traditions, morals, and beliefs eroded over the course of centuries due to colonialism and other forms of invasive outsider interference. Apart from dangerous or reportable situations, we must respect the differences of others by making a commitment to let a person choose how and from whom they get support.

Culturally astute counselors will recognize the longstanding tradition of trusting pastors as problem-solvers. They will appreciate the historic role of The Black Church as the place to go for every sort of help and support needed. Most importantly, they will respect the beliefs that make mental health and spiritual health synonymous and will not invalidate or devalue a client's belief system. Instead, they will allow each client to be guided by their convictions while asking if the client is interested in learning more about the brain's role in emotional distress. After all, this kind of psychoeducational reminder that the brain is a physical *organ* can be transformative.

NOTES

1. Albert A. Goodson, *We've Come This Far By Faith*, vinyl recording (Manna Music, Inc., 1956).

2. Albert A. Goodson, "We've Come This Far by Faith," Hymnary.org, accessed April 8, 2023, https://hymnary.org/text/dont_be_discouraged_when_troubles.

3. "The 2020 Census of American Religion," PRRI, June 2, 2022, https://www.prri.org/research/2020-census-of-american-religion. This note applies to the entire paragraph.

4. "Religious Landscape Study: Racial and Ethnic Composition," Pew Research Center's Religion & Public Life Project (Pew Research Center, 2014), https://www.pewresearch.org/religion/religious-landscape-study/racial-and-ethnic-composition.

5. Robert Joseph Taylor et al., "Black and White Differences in Religious Participation: A Multisample Comparison," *Journal for the Scientific Study of Religion* 35, no. 4 (December 1996): 403, https://doi.org/10.2307/1386415.

6. Federal Emergency Management Agency (FEMA), "Engagement Guidelines: Black Church Protestant Leaders, FEMA.org, accessed April 8, 2023, https://www.fema.gov/sites/default/files/2020-03/fema_faith-communities_black-church-protestant-leaders_1.pdf.

7. John J. Carey, "Black Theology: An Appraisal of the Internal and External Issues," *Theological Studies* 33, no. 4 (December 1972): 684–97. https://doi.org/10.1177/004056397203300403.

8. Carey, "Black Theology," 687.

9. W.E.B. Du Bois, *The Negro Church: Report of a Social Study made under the Direction of Atlanta University; Together with the Proceedings of the Eighth Conference for the Study of the Negro Problems, Held at Atlanta University, May 26th, 1903* (Atlanta: The Atlanta University Press, 1903). https://docsouth.unc.edu/church/negrochurch/dubois.html; Sterling Stuckey, "W. E. B. Du Bois: Black Cultural Reality and the Meaning of Freedom," in *Slave Culture: Nationalist Theory and the Foundations of Black America*, online ed. (Oxford Academic, 2013), 275–339.

10. Pew Research Center, "Religious Landscape Study."

11. Samir Abi, "Metaphysical Explanations," D+C, June 12, 2019, https://www.dandc.eu/en/article/west-africa-traditional-or-religious-practices-are-often-preferred-method-treating-mental#:~:text=Most%20Africans%20view%20mental%20disturbances,of%20a%20mentally%20ill%20person.

12. Abi, "Metaphysical Explanations," 2.

13. Thomas G. Plante, "Religion Has a Public Relations Problem: Integrating Evidence-Based Thinking into Clinical Practice," *Spirituality in Clinical Practice*, 2022, https://doi.org/10.1037/scp0000292.

14. Plante, "Religion Has."

15. Plante, "Religion Has."

16. Richard M. Ryan and Edward L. Deci, *Self-Determination Theory* (New York: Guilford Publications, 2017).

17. Plante, "Religion Has."

18. Pew Research Center, "Religious Landscape Study.."

19. Ann W. Nguyen, "Religion and Mental Health in Racial and Ethnic Minority Populations: A Review of the Literature," *Innovation in Aging* 4, no. 5 (August 2020): 3, https://doi.org/10.1093/geroni/igaa035.

20. William R. Miller and Stephen Rollnick, *Motivational Interviewing: Preparing People for Change* (New York: Guilford Press, 2002).

21. Elizabeth D. Kilmer et al., "Differential Early Termination Is Tied to Client Race/Ethnicity Status.," *Practice Innovations* 4, no. 2 (June 25, 2019): 88–98, https://doi.org/10.1037/pri0000085.

22. Derald Wing Sue et al., *Counseling the Culturally Diverse Theory and Practice* (Hoboken, NJ: Wiley, 2019).

CHAPTER 13

Black Resilience

Resilience is not about being able to bounce back like nothing has happened.
Resilience is your consistent resistance to giving up.

—JANNA CACHOLA

RESILIENCE: THE ABILITY TO REBOUND FROM ADVERSITY AND BE strengthened by the experience.[1] Another definition says resilience is "*the dynamic process that leads to positive adaptations within the context of significant adversity*"[2] (emphasis added). In the simplest terms, resilience is a long-term positive response to a negative situation. It is a quality by which a person is able to withstand hardship and recover from it well. Resilience is especially salient for coping with racial trauma. Research shows that African Americans with greater levels of resilience also have significantly greater psychological well-being, as evidenced by lower depressive and anxiety symptoms, less frequent suicide ideation, and more life satisfaction.[3]

In earlier chapters, we established that the well-being of Black Americans is generally explored from a deficit perspective rather than from a strength perspective. Black people are presumed to need resilience support. Unfortunately, little attention has been given to the fact that Black people in the United States have collectively demonstrated a consistent capacity to overcome a wide range of social, economic, and environmental challenges from enslavement to the present day. While injustice has taken a toll and claimed lives, there is wide variation in outcomes for Blacks in America, which suggests that individually and collectively, Black people possess and effectively use significant resources for resilience.[4]

Generally speaking, resiliency definitions lack consideration for the burden of the *ongoing* nature of historical, intergenerational, and race-based trauma. While every family experiences a range of painful events, many Black families have carried more than their share of adversities resulting from discrimination; wealth gaps; health care disparities; and systemic, institutional, and interpersonal racism. These wounds are not single events from which one can heal and put the proverbial past behind them. Racism poses constant concerns and imposes unjustifiable experiences of victimization. From national policy to interpersonal relationships, African Americans and other Black people are chronically confronted with exposure to racist rhetoric and disadvantages that have well-documented—and negative—health impacts.[5]

Nonetheless, African Americans and other Black people continue to individually and collectively overcome and bounce back from a broad range of adversities and major traumatic incidents. Exclusive discussions about disparities without conversations about resilience can depict African Americans as weak and vulnerable. Too often, reports suggest that "being Black" is a risk factor for numerous medical diagnoses and adverse outcomes because of some inherent and unmanageable risk. In reality, Black/African American people are strong and resilient. Racism is the risk factor, not race.

By its definition, resilience is determined by two factors. First, resilience involves a threat or exposure to a traumatic event or other significant adversity. Second, resilience is characterized by responses that are understood as healthy adaptations. A monocultural approach suggests that a resilient person must learn from their experience and move forward with positive emotions and coping skills to live a relatively happy "forever after" life. Despite its widespread acceptance, this conceptualization of resilience further stigmatizes and even pathologizes many Black Americans.

Seeing Resilience Through a Culturally Responsive Lens

A just and fair assessment of Black American resilience requires exploring capabilities in context rather than giving a diagnosis and focusing on perceived deficits in coping.[6] Wendy Sims-Schouten and Patricia Gilbert make the point that the current definition of resilience needs to be revisited and retooled because White middle class voices have defined resiliency concepts like "coping mechanisms," "positive emotions," and "successful traits."[7] In turn, racialized groups are othered and further oppressed.

Society's definition of resilience protects predominantly White interests from facing Black anger and assertiveness. As counselors, we should have a big problem with that. Resilience must be defined through a culturally responsive lens. The call to re-envision the concept of resilience among Black Americans must ring as a loud and clear alarm and must include the strengths that undergird Black resilient living. Gregory et al. cite Hollingsworth with this important observation about cultural sensitivity in determining resilience:

> The application of resilience theory to Black families requires that we consider both the adversity confronting them as individual families and as members of a racial minority and the qualities by which many are able to thrive and prosper in spite of the adversity.[8]

What, then, does it mean for a chronically marginalized and historically oppressed race of people to demonstrate resilience? The answer is in their historical narrative: They have already demonstrated resilience. They have survived. They have not given up.

Whatever the form of Black resistance, it demonstrates Black resilience!

The resilience Black Americans employ is a significant protective factor against adversity, and their psychological hardiness helps them maintain two important beliefs: (1) stressful situations will be manageable and (2) they, themselves, are capable of recovering.[9] With their ability to withstand adversity, they experience a strong sense of empowerment and greater coping capacity for stressful events.[10]

RESISTANCE AS RESILIENCE

Beyond positive emotions and coping mechanisms, Sims-Schouten and Gilbert recognize that resistance can also represent a healthy expression of resilience. They offer commentary that "resilience can also mean 'resistance,' i.e., resisting bad treatment and racism, as well as reflecting agency, identity and ownership of one's own life and choices within this. Reframing resilience thus means taking account of multifaceted and interactive effects of personal, material, institutional and political factors that impact on behaviour, wellbeing and resilience, as well as acknowledging that the way in which 'behaviour' is received is by default flawed, if this is largely informed by an oppressive White middle-class viewpoint."[11]

Resistance is viewed as a threat when it challenges status quo systems. Consider the acts of resistance on the part of African Americans. All of these are expressions of Black resilience:

1600s–1800s: Numerous rebellions and insurrections occur on ships and on plantations.

1850–1863: The Underground Railroad helps approximately 70,000 slaves resist and escape slavery.

May 17, 1954: A legal fight results in the US Supreme Court outlawing school segregation in *Brown v. Board of Education.*

September 3, 1955: Mamie Till insisted on having an open casket viewing and funeral service for her fourteen-year-old son, Emmett Till. Mamie went against the advice of many people and showed the world the horrific mutilation of her son's body perpetrated by the racists who kidnapped and murdered him in Money, Mississippi.

December 1, 1955: Rosa Parks is arrested in Montgomery, Alabama, for refusing to give up her seat on a bus to a White man.

December 5, 1955–November 13, 1956: African Americans walked and car-pooled for over eleven months in a city-wide bus boycott in Montgomery, Alabama. Their resistance led to a Supreme Court ban on segregated seating.

September 24–25, 1957: Resistance and public outcry result in President Eisenhower ordering federal troops to enforce school desegregation in Little Rock, Arkansas. Personally guarded by soldiers from the National Guard soldiers and the Army's 101st Airborne, the Little Rock Nine began regular class attendance at Central High School in Little Rock, Arkansas.

February 1, 1960: Black students from North Carolina Agricultural and Technical College stage sit-ins at a "Whites only" lunch counter in Greensboro, North Carolina.

April 16, 1960: The Student Nonviolent Coordinating Committee (SNCC) is founded to promote youth involvement in the Civil Rights Movement.

November 14, 1960: Six-year-old Ruby Bridges, escorted by four federal marshals, was the first Black child to integrate the all-white William Frantz Elementary School in Louisiana.

December 5, 1960: Resistance, public outcry, and legal battles result in the Supreme Court outlawing segregation in bus terminals.

January 6, 1961: The University of Georgia is desegregated after a federal judge orders that two African American students be admitted; White students jeer, "Two, four, six, eight, we don't want to integrate."

May 14, 1961: Freedom Riders are attacked in Alabama while testing compliance with bus desegregation laws.

May 21, 1961: Federal Marshals are sent to protect civil rights activists threatened by a mob in Montgomery, Alabama.

April 1, 1962: Civil rights groups join forces to launch voter registration drives.

August 28, 1963: Twenty-five thousand Americans march on Washington for civil rights.

June 20, 1964: Freedom Summer brings one thousand young civil rights volunteers to Mississippi.

July 2, 1964: The Civil Rights Act of 1964 was signed into law by President Lyndon Johnson, prohibiting discrimination in public places, providing for the integration of schools and other public facilities, and making employment discrimination illegal. It was the most sweeping civil rights legislation since Reconstruction.

March 7, 1965: Marchers at the Edmund Pettus Bridge in Selma, Alabama, risk their lives on Bloody Sunday for voting rights.

March 25, 1965: The civil rights march from Selma to Montgomery is completed.

July 9, 1965: Congress passes the Voting Rights Act of 1965.

2013: Three Black women, Alicia Garza, Patrisse Cullors, and Opal Tometi, organize the Black Lives Matter Movement to address unequal treatment and oppression and to demand an end to police brutality because the lives of Black people are just as important as those of others.

Yes, that is a history of necessary resistance, and it is evidence of the resilient spirit within African American and other Black communities.

There are countless other examples too substantial to name. When Black people resist oppression, they are refusing to give up, refusing to be overtaken by treacherous bigotry and hatred, and refusing to be controlled by unjust systems. When Black people resist injustice, they are engaging in a dynamic process to speak hope into their future days and the experiences of future generations.

But every act of resilience and resistance is not televised. Most acts of resistance are in the day-to-day commitments and sacrifices that individual citizens make in support of equity or personal betterment.

Resistance is in resigning from a job where inclusivity is not valued.

Resistance is holding people accountable for microaggressions against members of BIPOC communities.

Resistance is in not patronizing companies whose business practices exploit or harm BIPOC lives, even if patronizing another business is less convenient or less expensive.

Resistance is in accompanying an elderly friend or family member to the doctor to challenge medical racism when you have reason to question equitable care.

Resistance is when young Black boys attempt to advocate for themselves—in the only way they know how—against bias in the classroom, but they are labeled as uncooperative, oppositional, and difficult to manage. I call it resistance because oftentimes, the students are simply attempting to confront the disciplinary disparities and prejudicial treatment they observe. I call it resilience because their self-advocacy is an attempt to influence changes in their environment.

Counselors must pay attention to behavioral changes in counseling such as clients not doing their homework between sessions, becoming uncharacteristically combative, missing or arriving late for appointments, resisting the counselor's direction in therapy, or shifting from active to minimal participation in the therapeutic dialogue. It is easy to label the client as non-compliant, but the client might be taking a self-advocacy stance—in the best way they know how. The counselor holds the responsibility for asking if there has been an offense or race rupture in the therapeutic relationship, and then to invite dialogue that promotes mending and growth for both parties.

Sometimes, resistance is shown by breaking barriers and moving forward. At other times resistance is demonstrated by walking away. Whatever the form of Black resistance, it demonstrates Black resilience!

Notes

1. W. Henry Gregory, et al., "Black Family Resilience: An Introduction to Enriched Structural Family Therapy." *Urban Social Work* 3, no. 1 (May 2019): 51–69, doi: 10.1891/2474-8684.3.1.51.

2. Wendy Sims-Schouten and Patricia Gilbert, "Revisiting 'Resilience' in Light of Racism, 'Othering' and Resistance," *Race & Class* 64, no. 1 (April 2022): 84–94, https://doi.org/10.1177/03063968221093882.

3. Ijeoma Julia Madubata, "Racial Trauma, Psychological Well-Being, and the Moderating Effect of Resilience in African American Adults," (PhD. diss., University of Houston, 2022).

4. Herman A. Taylor, Tulani Washington-Plaskett, and Arshed A. Quyyumi, "Perspective: Black Resilience—Broadening the Narrative and the Science on Cardiovascular Health and Disease Disparities," *Ethnicity & Disease* 30, no. 2 (April 23, 2020): 365–68.

5. Taylor, Washington-Plaskett, and Ouyyumi, "Perspective: Black Resilience."

6. Gregory, et al., "Black Family Resilience."

7. Sims-Schouten and Gilbert, "Revisiting 'Resilience,'" 84.

8. Gregory, et al., "Black Family Resilience."

9. George A. Bonanno, "Loss, Trauma, and Human Resilience: Have We Underestimated the Human Capacity to Thrive after Extremely Aversive Events?" *American Psychologist* 59, no. 1 (2004): 20–28, https://doi.org/10.1037/0003-066X.59.1.20.

10. Sadhbh Joyce et al., "Road to Resilience: A Systematic Review and Meta-Analysis of Resilience Training Programmes and Interventions," *BMJ Open* 8, no. 6 (June 14, 2018), https://doi.org/10.1136/bmjopen-2017-017858.

11. Sims-Schouten and Gilbert, "Revisiting 'Resilience,'" 84.

About the Author

LaVerne Hanes Collins, Ph.D., LPC (GA), LCMHC (NC), NCC, ACS, is a licensed counselor, author, trainer, keynote speaker, and workshop facilitator, in addition to serving as an adjunct instructor/lecturer and advisor for university graduate-level counseling programs.

Dr. Collins has a passion for understanding the intersection of clinical and societal issues related to race, faith, culture, and trauma. She specializes in the areas of multicultural counseling competencies, treatment needs, and disparities among racialized and minoritized groups, organizational inclusivity, and faith-based competencies in mental health.

Dr. Collins is the owner of New Seasons Counseling, Training, and Consulting LLC. She is established as a Diversity Trainer and Consultant in behavioral health, medicine, education, and business. She is known, not only as a therapist and trainer but also as a coach and mentor who helps counselors across the nation develop specializations in multicultural mental health training and consulting.

In addition to her first book, *The Fruit of Your Pain: Experiencing Spiritual Renewal Through Seasons of Struggle*, Dr. Collins has published several works, in textbooks, encyclopedias, and trade publications, including a two-year series of articles titled "Honoring Diversity" in the American Counseling Association (ACA) monthly magazine *Counseling Today*. Collins is married and enjoys traveling and spending time with friends and family, especially her grandchildren, who affectionately call her "Lovie!"

www.ingramcontent.com/pod-product-compliance
Lightning Source LLC
Chambersburg PA
CBHW020000290326
41935CB00007B/245

* 9 7 8 1 4 7 5 8 6 7 5 7 2 *